short fat
chick to
marathon
Runner

KERRE WOODHAM

WITH GARETH BROWN

short fat chick to marathon *Runner*

HarperCollins*Publishers*

National Library of New Zealand Cataloguing-in-Publication
Woodham, Kerre.
Short fat chick to marathon runner / Kerre Woodham, Gareth
Brown.
ISBN 978-1-86950-670-4
1. Woodham, Kerre. 2. Marathon running—Training.
3. Physical fitness. 4. Weight loss. 5. Diet.
I. Brown, Gareth, 1979- II. Title.
613.7172—dc 22

First published 2008
Reprinted 2008 (four times)
Reprinted 2009 (twice)
HarperCollins*Publishers (New Zealand) Limited*
P.O. Box 1, Auckland

ISBN: 978 1 86950 670 4

Cover design by Matt Stanton
Cover photograph by Charlie Smith
Internal text design and typesetting by Springfield West
Printed by Griffin Press, Australia

70gsm Classic used by HarperCollins*Publishers* is a natural,
recyclable product made from wood grown in sustainable
forests. The manufacturing processes conform to the
environmental regulations in the country of origin, Finland.

To the Irishman, my daughter, the dog, and all those who ran with me, metaphorically and literally, on this journey.

contents

chapter one

The midlife crisis and the marathon

With the benefit of hindsight it was inevitable that I'd run a marathon in my forties. It's a total cliché — middle-aged woman, midlife crisis, run a marathon — and my life has been a series of clichés. From good Catholic girl, to very bad Catholic girl, to hard-drinking journo, to suburban wife and mother, to teetotalling dairy-free couscous muffin-maker par excellence. Why wouldn't I run a marathon? Although halfway through my forty-first year, I thought it would be more likely that I would sell our comfortable Grey Lynn cottage, quit my job on NewsTalkZB and head for the West Coast with the Irishman and the Border collie in tow.

I was unsettled, bored to sobs with life in general and desperate for a new project. A dear friend had died six months previously, my daughter was leaving school at the end of the year and there was no denying that I was getting old. My skin was creasing into folds — where there used to be one line when I bent my arm, there were now about six.

My weight has always fluctuated between healthy and fat, and I was definitely in a fat phase with no idea how to get out of it. And what is it with hair when you hit your forties? It greys, sure — I was prepared for that. But why does it suddenly corkscrew out of your follicles and do mad things to your eyebrows? And why does it suddenly appear on your thighs? My thighs have never been the favourite part of my body, but hairy thighs are truly hideous. My body was packing up and it appeared my mind was following fast.

Midway through that year, I can remember standing in the middle of our lounge and wailing 'I just want to run away!' And I did. I was quite serious. I wanted to run away from my job, my house, my responsibilities and my life.

The long-suffering Irishman sensed that trouble was looming. He looked up from the television, pressed the mute button, and asked, 'If you're going to be running away, will you be taking me, now?'

I appraised him, sitting there, handsome and infuriating and solid, and decided he might as well be my one constant. 'Yes, I suppose so,' I snapped back. 'It's utterly pointless training up a new man now.'

'Good,' he replied equably, and turned the sound back up.

I suppose some women have affairs when they hit their midlife crises, but really, how do they do it? A breathless passion-filled encounter with a young man sounds fine in theory, but the practicalities are overwhelming when you think about it. First, there's finding a willing partner in moral crime, then there's the actual mechanics of it — getting your gear off, and exposing your failing flesh to another set of eyes. Eyes that haven't got used to the gradual decline of your form over a period of years. These would be fresh eyes. Eyes that have lingered over bodies far younger and firmer than yours. Eyes that might be clouded with lust briefly, but in the cold, harsh post-coital light of day would be terribly unforgiving.

I remember going to a function where I was one of the masters of ceremony. It was a black tie function and there were going to be various luminaries there, so it was one of those nights where I'd pulled out all the stops. I'd had my hair and make-up professionally done, I'd had the spray tan, and I was in one of my most fabulous frocks, an Adrienne Winkelmann with a plunging neckline, a bit of a train at the back and slashed to the thigh at the front. So I looked about as good as a girl can look.

At the end of the night, a young man approached me, shoved me against a table with his crotch, and with all the sincerity a boy can muster with eighteen tequila slammers inside him, told me I was '(expletive deleted) hot' and that he had a room downstairs and should he upgrade to a suite? This was followed up with a suggestive pelvic thrust. I thanked him for his attentions but pointed out that I was nearly forty and he looked to be in his twenties. He told me that was OK, he digged older chicks (quote unquote) and how about it?

I looked at the gorgeous young thing, and thought if I didn't have the Irishman at home, I'd let the cheeky whippersnapper take me downstairs and let nature follow its course. Then in the morning, as he lay there poleaxed with the pain of his hangover, I would whip open the curtains and let the brutal sunlight illuminate the room.

The magic of the heated rollers that had transformed my hair into tumbling blonde tendrils would have dissipated, the false eyelashes would be clinging to my cheeks like drunken spiders, the artfully applied make-up would be all over the pillows, exposing the flaws of my near forty-year-old face, the hideously expensive push-up bra would be dangling off a lightshade and my poor old boobs would be hanging around my hips, and the fake tan would have rubbed off, leaving my pallid white skin to shine through.

And if he was really lucky, there would be the glint of an errant grey pubic hair in the harsh light. That would teach the young pup to hit on older women, I thought to myself, but as I looked into his drink-befuddled eyes, I realised it was too cruel a life lesson to be giving to such a young man, so I gave him a reprieve instead and told him to find someone his own age to play with and off he lurched, little realising how close he'd come to making one of the more monumental mistakes of his young life.

So an affair was simply out of the question, but how then to resolve the midlife crisis without making a grand gesture I would probably live to regret.

The answer came with a phone call. I love the phone. All my working life the phone has delivered to me fabulous propositions and possibilities. The first time I ever travelled to Europe was thanks to a phone call.

I never thought I'd make it to Europe before I turned sixty, but there I was languishing in a Wellington restaurant, taking a hiatus from the world of media — strictly speaking,

I think the media was taking a break from me — and the phone went and there it was: the offer to travel to London and Rome, presenting a TV travel show. There've been plenty of phone calls like that over the years, so when the phone goes, I'm the first to pick it up.

Dorothy Parker, the fabulous American writer, used to groan theatrically when the phone rang or there was a knock at the door: 'What fresh hell is this?' But not me. No, no, no. The phone has delivered some amazing opportunities into my home and my life and, yet again, the phone was about to deliver. Although on the face of it, this didn't seem like much of an opportunity.

This time, when the phone rang, it was Antonia, one of the lovely girls from Pead PR, one of the top PR companies in the country. She had a client, she said, Regal Salmon, who would like to sponsor me for the Auckland Marathon. They wanted someone high-profile, who was a good fit for Regal's target market (household shoppers) and someone thirty-five plus. I would get five grand, either for myself or for a charity. They would pay all my setting-up expenses for a month, and then for a trainer once a week after that, as well as feeding me up on all the salmon I could eat.

A marathon! Me? Run a marathon! I was overweight, middle-aged, and although I'd jogged a bit when I was younger, the most I'd ever run was round the block. I couldn't run a marathon. I said I'd talk it over with the family and call her back. A marathon.

I had a friend who used to run marathons. She loved the training, loved the time out on the streets, having time to herself to just think and run. We all thought she was mad. Another friend of mine had run the Rotorua Marathon years ago, but she never ran another one. And I have an aunt and uncle who run marathons. When we used to stay with them down in Christchurch, they would disappear for two-hour training runs in the scorching heat of a Canterbury nor'wester. Barking. And that's it. The sum total of my knowledge of marathon runners. However, the Irishman and my daughter thought it was a great idea.

'You need a challenge,' they said.

'You're bored and restless.'

'You'd lose weight,' my daughter said.

And that was a big spur. I'd lost a lot of weight a couple of years ago, through the liver cleansing diet and regular kickboxing sessions, but gradually the bad food habits had crept back in and my trainer had gone overseas, so the exercise had gone by the board. I was 73 kilos — and that was 13 kilos more than I really needed to be.

My clothes didn't fit me any more. I was looking like a plump hausfrau and I wasn't ready to be one of those. Besides, the idea of testing my body really appealed to me. It's always been a functional body, as opposed to an aesthetically pleasing one. It works. It seldom breaks down. I haven't had much trouble with it, despite giving it a fair old caning in my twenties. I'd enjoyed kickboxing, mainly because I could appreciate my body for what it could do — jump, kick, punch — rather than grizzle about what it couldn't do.

OK, so I wasn't elfin or gamine, but I was strong and powerful. And I was curious to know whether my mind was strong enough to run a marathon. Even though I knew very little about marathon running, I'd picked up enough to know that running is 90 per cent a mind game. It's having the willpower to put on your shoes and get out there and start running. So in the absence of any other bright ideas on how to get over my ennui, I rang Antonia and agreed to run the Auckland Marathon.

I met the lovely people from Regal at Pead PR's Newmarket offices. It was all a bit daunting. The last guy they'd sponsored — Dom, the breakfast host on the Edge — did all the training and half an hour into the marathon had a total collapse and was carted off to hospital for a lifesaving operation. They were hoping the same thing wouldn't happen to me. As indeed was I.

I decided to donate the money to the Cystic Fibrosis Association of New Zealand, mainly because I'd heard Tracey Richardson speak — she has two kids with the disorder and she transformed her life by running the Hawaiian Ironman to raise funds for the CFA. Inspirational? Oh my word, she is. In fact, if you want to change your life, put down this book and go out and get hers. Come back to me. I'll still be here.

Inspired by Tracey, I'd actually tried to win some money for the CFA by naming them as my charity in an invitational poker tournament at the Christchurch Casino earlier in the year, but I'd bummed out. I felt I owed the organisation. Now I could finally make a significant donation. But that was only if I finished the marathon and we were working against the clock. By the time everyone involved had signed off the necessary paperwork, it was the middle of May. The marathon was the end of October.

Five months to get me from couch potato to marathon runner. I knew it was going to involve quite a bit of work, but really. Come on. Oprah had run a marathon, for God's sake. Blind people run them all the time. I seemed to recall a one-legged man running the London Marathon. So I was a little overweight. So I'd never run before. How hard could it be? I was about to find out.

GAZ

I remember being on a course at Les Mills when my boss, Norm Phillips, came into the room and pulled me aside.

'I've got a client for you. She's a talkback host, needs to run a marathon and I think you're the man for the job.'

I thought, no probs . . . been done before.

He handed me the details: Kerre Woodham; wants to run Auckland Marathon 2006.

My first thoughts were: Blonde curly hair, famous for being candid, more than a handful and was on *Fair Go*. I used to watch it with my family. My mum was a big fan of Kerre and carries a few of the same traits. She's a straight shooter, tells you how it is and doesn't like me bastardising my given name Gareth by changing it to Gaz. I knew from the start we were going to get along just fine.

My second thought was, there must be a printing error. Auckland Marathon 2006! At that stage we had 23 weeks to go! As a trainer, you always want the odds stacked in your favour. A history of fitness in the chosen discipline, a motivated, dedicated and enthusiastic client who has the wallet to pay for it ('cause I'm not cheap!) and a realistic time frame. At least a couple of boxes were ticked!

I met with Kerre on 20 May 2006. It was 9 a.m. on a lovely Saturday morning. Kerre is an attractive woman who really knows how to present herself, but that day she was looking a little rough around the edges. A few too many Grey Lynn luncheons had obviously taken their toll.

Many people who watch a great event like the Taupo Ironman get an urge to give up work for a year, go on the benefit, and train day and night until they get to push themselves to the brink of oblivion. That urge normally fades after 24 hours, then it all settles down, reality sets in and it's back to the grind of a regular lifestyle.

For Kerre, the idea of running a marathon had obviously gone past the initial excitement phase and moved into reality. I was excited at this prospect. I mean, for Kerre to turn around to her family and announce that she was going to run the marathon and initiate a meeting must have taken some balls. What I was about to learn was that Kerre had never watched a marathon, let alone considered the distance. In her mind it was 22 km long and wouldn't be that hard! My excitement suddenly turned into a surge of nervousness!

chapter two

A pretty boy called Gaz

The first step was finding a trainer. And for a trainer, I went to Les Mills. I'd been a member at Les Mills ever since the iconic former *Nightline* presenter, Belinda Todd, had taken me under her well-toned bicep when I joined the TV3 crew fifteen years previously.

Belinda was a star — a gorgeous, utterly unorthodox redhead who turned television on its head when she exploded onto the screen back in the late eighties. Sitting squatly on the *Fair Go* set over at Television New Zealand all those years ago, I loathed her. She was everything I wasn't. Beautiful, wilful, outrageous and loved by the critics. Just eighteen short months later, I was working with her, having run away from a secure job with the national broadcaster, the city I called home and a relationship. And I adored her.

Belinda's naughtiness was all an act. In actual fact, she was a desperately shy serial monogamist with a passion for physical fitness. She insisted that I come along with her to the aerobics classes she taught, and before I knew it, I was a Les Mills member and a gym junkie. I had never looked better than when Belinda whipped me into shape and, over the years, I had kept up my membership at the gym, even though Belinda was living in LA and months went by between my visits to the gym. So it was to the team at Les Mills that I turned now that I needed to find a trainer to get me across the line of the Auckland Marathon. I put in a call to Norm, the gym manager.

'Norm,' I said, 'I'm going to be running the Auckland Marathon for charity. I need a trainer — the company sponsoring me will pay for him. And I need a *real* trainer — I don't want some pretty boy who's going to tell me I'm fabulous.' Even the best gyms have pretty boys, and Les Mills was no exception. When I was going through my dairy-free, teetotalling, couscous muffin-making phase, I was also kickboxing three times a week. And while I was kicking the crap out of my staunch Iranian trainer, I was infuriated by the pretty PTs, who would be checking themselves out in the mirrors while their forty-something female clients sweated away on Swiss balls. It seemed disrespectful and I'd be buggered if I had to rely on one of those to get me through. Still, I suppose we all get through our midlife crises in our own ways and if these pretty boys enabled a middle-aged housewife to endure menopause without shooting herself or members of her family, then so much the better.

Norm assured me that he would find the right man for the job and within 24 hours he'd called me back with a name and a time to meet my new trainer. His name, said Norm, was Gaz and he was just back from a few years working in England. He'd been a triathlete in his day and he'd just started with Les Mills. I was to meet him at 10 on Saturday morning.

The first meeting didn't go all that well. I don't think either of us was terrifically impressed. Who calls themselves Gaz, for God's sake? He was exactly what I'd told Norm I didn't want. He was young, cute and his name was Gaz. Could it have been any worse?

I was hung-over, given that it was the morning after Friday night and I'd started drinking again. For seven years the Irishman and I had forsworn alcohol, for reasons I shan't go into. That's a book in itself. Suffice to say, we both really, really needed to take a break from the booze for a while.

And so we did. For seven years we didn't touch a drop and then slowly, from my fortieth birthday, we crept back into the liquor cabinet. And we were OK. We certainly were nowhere near as hideous as we had been, but we were drinking. And it would have probably been a better idea to run a marathon during the dry years. But there it was. I was drinking and I was about to begin training for a marathon — if I could convince this young whippersnapper in front of me to take me on as a client. Because he was looking at me with cold, clinical eyes, and it was clear he was finding me wanting.

My recollection of our initial conversation went something like this:

Gaz: You're going to have to drop some weight before you start serious running otherwise you're going to get injured.

Kerre (chin up, refusing to accept any criticism; won't be told what to do by someone young enough to be her little brother): I don't want to lose weight. I like having tits and an arse. I really don't want a runner's body.

Gaz: Well, you're not going to be able to run a marathon with the body you have.

And then a little later as Gaz tried to drive home just what was involved in running a marathon:

Gaz: You do realise this is an enormous undertaking.

Kerre: Oh, for heaven's sake! How hard can it be to run two and a half hours?

Gaz (icily): That's the world record. If you do it in under five hours, I'll be amazed.

Some people might have taken offence to that opening gambit, but I've always liked straight shooting — even if the thought of running for five hours turned my bowels to water. Gaz wasn't being unkind, he was just telling it like it was, and I like that in a person. The fact that I walked the dog forty minutes to an hour each day was a bonus. Gaz said that if you're a walker, generally you can be trained to be a runner. But he had to find out whether under all my flab, my body was strong enough to take all the punishment that would be involved in taking me from dog-walker to marathon runner. We agreed to meet later in the week when he would do an initial assessment before deciding whether I was up to the job or not.

Part of that assessment involved visiting a chiropractor, Iain Wood. A former rugby player, Iain looks after plenty of sportspeople and has a good understanding of the human form, in a chiropractic kind of way. He sent me along for a spinal X-ray to make sure my underworked body would be up for the challenge of a marathon and after he'd cast his eye over my bones, he gave me the all clear. Although there'd be quite a bit of work involved, there was no structural reason why I couldn't be trained to run 42 kilometres. I was on my way.

My first run was just 10 minutes long. That was pretty much a run around the block. I was accustomed to walking the Border collie for at least forty minutes a day, so a quiet ten-minute jog didn't faze me. I spent longer working out what to wear than I did pounding the pavements. It's a tricky one for a first-time, overweight female runner. You want to hide as much of your body as possible and yet you want to be comfortable. Those freaks of human nature who have 3 per cent body fat are sorted. Singlets and those little nylon shorts are ideal for both men and women, and some of the women don't even have to worry about harnessing their hooters. For those of us who are yet to attain the ultimate runner's physique, it's a little more difficult.

I had some old running shorts from the Belinda Todd/ *Nightline* years a decade ago, but they would be hopeless. There was a bloke at school who was nicknamed Wubs because his thighs rubbed together. I didn't want to be known as the Wubs Woodham of the wunning world because of my thighs — and besides, chafing's bloody painful. I also discounted board shorts — what's comfortable to run in for an hour can become jolly uncomfortable after two and undoubtedly unbearable after four.

Tops were also an issue — the manufacturers don't cut them long and I didn't want one that rode up. I opted for one of my Irishman's T-shirts and Lycra leggings. The

T-shirt would cover my stomach and the Lycra leggings came to my knees, so there wouldn't be too much in the way of thigh exposed. And off I went.

The ten-minute run wasn't difficult, but I knew from the training diary that Gaz had given me that the runs were going to become progressively longer and presumably tougher. The diary stretched out a month ahead — it seemed incredible to me that within three weeks I'd be running an hour. But I'd put my faith in Gaz and he in me, so I followed the training programme religiously.

From the ten-minute run, I progressed to a thirty-five minute run around the block. In the early days, I used to be a carbon Big Foot, as I'd drive the route I intended to run counting the kilometres on the odometer. Although Gaz had me running by time, rather than distance, as a newbie runner you do become a little obsessed about how far you've come — and, indeed, how much further you have to go. Later I discovered www.mapmyrun.com and that's a very handy little website for all runners. It does indeed map your run from start to finish — provided you run along streets and roads. It's not so great mapping off-road routes. And remember to ask the computer to give you kilometres, not miles. I almost cried when I saw how few ks I'd burned up until I realised I was getting the distance in miles.

The first time I ran the thirty-five minute circuit I felt like my work was done. Surely no-one in the field of human endeavour could be expected to run further than that. But Gaz had me run it a couple more times and then, once I'd become blasé about my short jaunt around the block, he set me to running forty minutes. We were building a strong working relationship. Once he saw I was willing to follow his instructions to the letter and once I realised he knew exactly what he was doing and there was a reason for everything we were doing, we trusted one another and that trust built into a mutual respect and liking.

I was even willing to accept there was a reason for the Devil's Staircase — a sheer vertical set of stairs going from just past Victoria Park to Herne Bay. I'd run up them as fast as I possibly could and Gaz would time me. I hated that part of our training, but once Gaz had patiently explained what muscles I'd be using, how they would be strengthened by that particular exercise and that they would be built up more quickly that way than by doing any other exercise, I could grit my teeth and get through it. Although I was very glad when we moved on from that particular aspect of my training!

Our first goal was the Woodbourne Half-marathon — Woodbourne being a tiny settlement just out of Blenheim. That was chosen for us because Regal Salmon wanted to show us around their operation based in Picton, just twenty minutes' drive away. The aim was to fly down, run the half, do a quick tiki tour of the company's salmon fishery and then fly home. Sounded like a plan, and it was good to have the half-marathon as a focus for training.

I can still remember my first one-hour run. I'd finished hosting my Sunday morning radio show and I came home, got into my running gear and headed out before the lure of lunch sidetracked me from my mission.

For me, the hardest part about running was — and still is — getting out the door. It usually takes me about two hours of intense negotiation with myself before I stop faffing around, inventing ever-more ludicrous reasons why I shouldn't run, and actually get myself out of the house and onto the streets. The first ten minutes are always hell, too, and for my inaugural 60-minute run, there was no exception. I creaked and groaned and ached and moaned to myself, but by the time I'd got the first couple of ks under my belt — or under my shoes — I was feeling a lot better. And finishing a run is a fabulous sensation. The smug feeling of virtue and a job well done lasts the entire day. And the buzz from achieving the milestone of my first 10 km, my one-hour run, was fabulous. If I felt this good after one hour, just imagine how fantastic I was going to feel after a marathon!

By this time, I'd progressed from wearing oversized T-shirts and long Lycra leggings to proper running shirts and short Lycra leggings. I couldn't yet run in shorts because the one pair I had were too short. I tried them once and the chafing I experienced was agony. When you've got fleshy thighs, they're going to rub together, so either put plenty of Vaseline on the wobbly bits or go for the Lycra leggings. While you're at it, smear some Vaseline on your nipples as well. Don't linger — keep your mind on the job in hand. The only thing worse than chafed thighs is chafed nipples. And this may seem like stating the obvious, but don't wear a G-string when you go for a run.

I should have known about the dangers of G-strings since my *Intrepid Journey* to Cambodia. I was one of the lucky New Zealanders chosen to front one of these fantastic travel shows and my trip was a breeze. Some of the poor presenters really suffered, but not me. Apart from one fateful trip by motorbike up to Bokor. We hired four local lads to take us up to the national park, as it was a good four hours away and inaccessible by car. Being a good Catholic girl, I'd never been on the back of a motorbike before, but I took to it like a duck to water. Bouncing along over dried riverbeds and felled trees and round winding tracks. It was fantastic. Except it was a long journey and my bum was getting really sore. Sorer by the hour. The motorbike was a trail bike with good suspension and I had plenty of natural padding, so I just put it down to the novelty of the situation. However, by the time we got to the huts at the top of the mountain, I could barely walk. I staggered into the bunkroom, followed by Jane the producer. I pulled up my skirt to reveal a blister the size of a bread and butter plate. I had been wearing a G-string — so much easier to wash and dry when you're travelling, but which should never, ever be worn on a motorbike. The bouncing and jouncing and rubbing over four hours had burned a potentially dangerous blister into the crack of my bum. Poor Jane gasped and said she really thought they should airlift me out — apparently blisters can be quite dangerous if they get infected. I was horrified. Imagine being known as the girl who'd had to be airlifted out of Cambodia because of the blister on her bum. I would probably appear as a gag on *Letterman*. I promised I would be fine and Jane doubtfully offered to slap a blister pack onto it, but really, there wasn't a lot you could do and there's only so much producers should have to do. So much for the glamour of television. I suffered — although not in silence — and learnt a valuable lesson: some activities are not meant for G-strings.

Riding on the back of a motorbike and training for a marathon are two activities where nana pants are required.

Make sure, too, that the running shirts are long enough to cover your tummy if you've got a flabby one. Some of those running shirts are made for people with the vital statistics of underfed whitebait. There's nothing worse than pounding along and having to hitch down your shirt with every stride. Apart, perhaps, from seeing women drive past, pity mingled with contempt in their eyes as they watch your lumbering progress. I know what they're thinking, because I used to think it too when I drove past overweight women running along the street. 'Oh dear. Bless. Oh well. At least she's out there, trying.' I had become an object of pity but don't let that put you off. Runner's smugness is a powerful antidote to pity.

One of my colleagues in Radio Sport, Brendan Telfer, hit me up when I got to work one day as I was nearing the end of my training.

'Saw you out running yesterday. Geez, you were making hard work of it.'

'It was a sixteen k run,' I responded icily. 'Actually, it *was* hard work.'

'It's people like you who give running a bad name,' he sniggered, heading off to his desk and earning my lifelong enmity. Not everyone's born a natural athlete. Of course it's more splendid to see a gifted and aesthetically beautiful athlete in full flight, but there are bugger-all of them around. I saw precious few of them in Grey Lynn. Most of us are imperfect, and support and encouragement is the civilised response to anyone taking up any sort of exercise, not sneering put-downs.

To be fair to Brendan, though, very few people thought me running a marathon was a good idea. When I decided to give up the booze, I got plenty of support and congratulations. When I decided to give up running restaurants and go back to radio, same again. People couldn't have been more pleased for me. But when I announced my decision to run a marathon, my friends and work colleagues looked at me as if I'd announced that from now on, I would live my life naked. There was mingled horror and awe. I had the support of my Irishman and my daughter — and without their support, I couldn't have even contemplated running the marathon. Marathon training takes up an awful lot of time — time that could be spent with the family. It feels awfully selfish sometimes as you head out on a two-hour run, leaving domestic chaos behind you. (It feels awfully good leaving the rest of the family to sort out the chaos, too!) There are ways to absolve your conscience though. I roped in the editor of the *New Zealand Herald*, Tim Murphy, to run the Auckland Marathon as well. He told me at a function we were both attending that he'd always wanted to run a marathon, but he felt he needed the impetus of running for a charity.

I became quite evangelical when I started running. Struggling with the handicap of running with the physique of a prop, I considered it a dreadful waste for anyone long and lean not to be out there running. Tim was one of those people blessed with a natural runner's body and once he'd admitted that running a marathon was a goal he'd always wanted to achieve, that was it. One of our company honchos was part of the group as the discussion was taking place and he told Tim he'd match Regal's sponsorship of me, dollar for dollar. And just like that, Tim was on the way to becoming a marathon runner. He was concerned about the amount of time he would be away from his lovely wife and young children, so he got around that by hiring his niece as a babysitter every Sunday when he went on his long runs and that way he got to train, and his wife got time to herself as well. Not a bad option if you can do it as a way of keeping your partner on side.

As the Woodbourne Half got closer and closer and my runs got longer, my friends started to realise I was serious. And so they swung in behind me with encouragement. The other trainers at the gym began taking an interest in Gaz and me, and started asking after our training. I think some of them wanted to see Gaz fall flat on his face. He was the new kid in town, there was quite a bit of media attention and his professional reputation was riding on getting the short fat blonde across the line. Most, though, were genuinely interested and wished us well. It was a good feeling.

GAZ

It has to be said from the onset, to run a marathon with no previous running experience takes certain credentials. In the first place, a marathon should not be run until a half-marathon has been completed. Depending on the structural condition of the body, the programme up to a marathon, including the half, can take anywhere from thirty-six weeks upwards.

I'll attempt to take you through the steps I would use to introduce a new client to running. Please be aware that this is just from my experience and has no scientific backing.

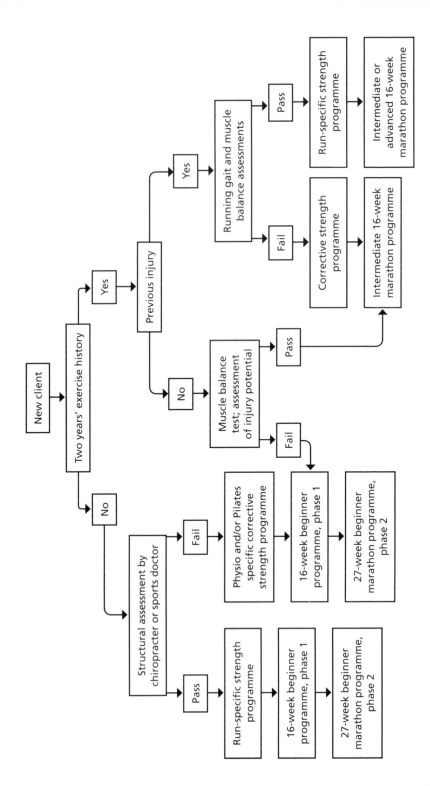

As you can imagine, Kerre did not fit very well into my flow chart! We had twenty-three weeks to go, she had no previous running experience and had accumulated years of abuse on her body — at a social level, not sporting!

At least we had a clean slate! To tell you the truth, Kerre had a large desire to complete a marathon. As much as she plays herself down, she has amazing drive, practises what she preaches and has an infectious enthusiasm. She's great fun to be around. I thought that if I could transfer her energy into running, then we'd be away. Another factor in her favour was that she walked her dog Toby every day. This proved to be one of her saving graces. If you want to run a marathon but you've got no solid sporting base to build from, then get walking as soon as possible. Work up to an hour a day, and then we can talk business.

chapter three

Running with Rats

I had always assumed that running was a solitary pursuit, but, in fact, it's very much a team sport. Sure, you're on your own when you're out there running. You're the one who has to put one foot in front of the other. But I found that running with a group can make all the difference as to whether or not you enjoy your training. I was lucky that an acquaintance of mine, Mary Lambie, was training for the New York Marathon, which was to be held the week after Auckland. The timing was perfect. I forget who contacted whom, but we spoke on the phone and Mary offered to run with me on Saturday mornings. I had worked with Mary when she hosted the *Good Morning* show on Television New Zealand. I was the sometime book reviewer and although I liked Mary, I hadn't spent much time socially with her. She was busy with three children under four, a husband, her media commitments and paying an Auckland mortgage. I was busy with university, a teenage daughter, my Irishman, my job on the radio and other speaking and writing jobs, and I too was paying an Auckland mortgage. It didn't leave us much time to chat over the teacups. But I was delighted to have someone to run long distances with and given that we lived in the same area, it made it most convenient. She introduced me to her two friends who were running New York as well. Lee was tiny and could run like the wind, and Lavina was young and gorgeous and could run fast too. It made for quite a good group. Although Lavina lived in Tauranga, she was often in Auckland through work commitments. The two speedy ones could head off with one another, while Mary and I brought up the rear.

I cannot stress how important it is to arrange to meet someone for your long runs, especially if, like me, you can talk yourself out of doing anything you don't want to do. When the alarm goes at 6.15 a.m. on Saturday morning and it's cold and dark and looking like rain, every fibre of your being screams at you to roll over, pull up the covers and go back to sleep. It is absolute madness to get up, put on running gear and head out onto the streets. There is simply no logical reason why anyone should do it. Your body knows this, your mind knows this, and without the impetus of an arranged meeting, it would be just too easy to put off the run for another time or another day. And that way lies failure. Knowing that somebody would be hanging around in the dark and the cold waiting for me provided me with a sufficient spur to get up and out the door.

Why run so early? Well, a number of reasons. You don't have to, of course. You can run at any time of the day or night. However, most marathons have 6 a.m. start times, so it's a good idea to get your body used to functioning at such an obscene hour. If your body knows to expect a banana and a gallon of water at 6 a.m., and to organise itself so that you don't have to madly find a loo in the middle of a run, so much the better. You can also enjoy the rest of the day without having the prospect of the long run hanging over you. I found I couldn't enjoy my Saturday unless the bloody run had been done. If you get the run out of the way first thing in the morning, it leaves you the rest of the day to enjoy yourself. And if you're up at dawn's crack, you're able to run for a couple of hours without inhaling buckets of exhaust fumes, as normal people aren't up and driving at 6 a.m. on a Saturday.

I used to be a normal person. The jobs I worked started late and finished later, and the only time I ever did mornings was when I was doing the walk of shame, apart from one brief stint as a breakfast host on an ill-fated radio station with the legendary radio jock, Kevin Black. That was an abject disaster. I'd crawl into work at 5.30 a.m., champagne glass in one hand, stilettos in the other, and entourage in tow. I didn't last long, but then neither did the radio station. So mornings and me don't really work, but that had to change during the lead-up to the marathon. It made sense to run early in the morning, and so I did. Less exhaust to breathe, fewer people around to see me in full flight. Call me shallow, call me vain, but I'd really rather not encounter people I know while I'm out running. They're sitting at an outside table at a trendy café, all chic and weekend casual, and I lumber past, scarlet-faced, frizzy-haired and bits of me in perpetual motion even after I come to a halt. Running is not a spectator sport when it's done by amateurs and I'd rather minimise contact with non-runners.

And I have to say that running in the early morning is fun. Not fun in any kind of easily understood or accepted way, but an activity that generates a sense of joy and wellbeing can be called fun, can't it? If anyone had told me back in my skanky, hard-drinking ho days that one Saturday morning I'd be jogging up Mount Eden, just as the day was breaking, I'd have rasped a smoker's laugh and poured another drink. But there is something utterly wonderful, in a masochistic, spot-the-girl-with-the-Catholic-education, self-flagellating kind of way about sweating and groaning to the top of Mount Eden, the pay-off for the pain being the 360-degree panorama of the city and the feeling of absolute triumph at knocking the bastard off. Auckland's beautiful when she's asleep, and so few of us get to see her like that. That's why most runners do their runs, especially their long runs, early in the morning.

I was also fortunate in finding the Titirangi Tunnel Rats. In my job as columnist for the *Herald on Sunday*, I'd mentioned that I had committed to running the Auckland Marathon. I received a lovely email from a chap called Andy, inviting me to join the YMCA runners on a Sunday morning. When I told him I couldn't run on Sunday mornings due to my radio show, he forwarded on the address of a woman from a Titirangi group that ran on Saturdays, suggesting that I join up with them. So one morning, when Mary was away, I drove out to the Titirangi public toilets to meet up with the Tunnel Rats.

The Rats are a group of real runners who've been running together in the Waitakeres for years. They've all run marathons, some of them have even won marathons, but fortunately I didn't know this when I drove out for that first run. Had I known the calibre of these runners, I would never have dared presume to run with them, which would have been a terrible shame because they were incredibly welcoming and running with this group was one of the perks of training for the marathon.

That first run was a long one that crawled up the hill from Titirangi towards Piha. We were following in the footsteps of the legendary running coach Arthur Lydiard, who used the hills of the Waitakere Ranges to condition his runners. It's long, slow and brutal and our conversational chat fell away as the hills got steeper heading towards the Waiatarua Fire Station. We got to the top, paused to regroup and drink from the tap and then we had to do it all over again. I could never, ever have done it on my own, but running with the group made it bearable.

It also meant that I could enjoy the team aspect of sport, albeit in an individualistic way. I've never been able to play team sport because of the hours I work, so it was great to be part of a group of people who enjoyed the same activity and enjoyed motivating and supporting one another. I remember when I first went out to Titirangi we were running along merrily and about 10 km in, we stopped.

'Why are we stopping?' I asked the lead chap.

'To wait for the others,' he replied.

'Why?' I asked, thinking we all knew where we were going and where we were going to end up. What was the point in hanging around?

'Because,' he said patiently, 'it keeps up morale and it's a nice thing to do.'

Right. Niceness. Goodness. Team spirit. Must get more of that. I blushed with shame, but thankfully my face was scarlet from the running so nobody noticed. I don't think.

I was able to join the Rats most Saturday mornings,

and their running support and advice was invaluable. As indeed were the running tracks. Up hill and down dale, the climbs were torturous but really helped to build condition. Hill work apparently is vital if you want to improve your stamina, but human nature being what it is — well, my nature being what it is, anyway — I would go out of my way to avoid long runs with too many hills. Running with the Rats meant that the horror of hills was diminished as the team alongside me provided moral support and meant that I couldn't just give up and walk. Again, blame it on that old human nature, but I couldn't walk and lose face amongst the group, even if my upward incline jog was at the same speed as a slow walk!

Still, as the Irishman is wont to say, patience and perseverance will get a snail to Jerusalem, and patience, perseverance and pride got me up the hills of the Waitakeres. It was also far more pleasant to run through native bush and along deserted roads than it was to battle the smog and exhaust fumes of inner-city Auckland. You feel virtuous when you run; you double the virtuosity when you're cantering along amidst beautiful native bush. It was thanks to the Titirangi Tunnel Rats, too, that the girls and I met Bruce Matthews, one of the longtime Rats, and a man who was to prove a vital component in my attempt to run the Auckland Marathon.

GAZ

There is great importance to running with a group. Not only from a social point of view, but also from the view of progressing in running, gaining reassurance and building running knowledge. You see, by running with a group or someone else you start to build yourself a 'business-like mind' for running. Running attracts a wide range of people, so you tend to get individuals from each of the different personality types. You can learn something from all of these and apply it to your running. For example, someone who has an organised type of personality will generally always run with structure to their programme and follow strict guidelines. They are great with splits and train with a heart-rate monitor. On the other hand, a practical type of personality will tend to run without a heart-rate monitor, and choose their distance and pace depending on how their body feels. They usually know some great running routes and will entertain you for hours while running.

We all know that to run a successful business you need to collect people around you who strengthen your weaknesses. The same is true of a running group — you can use those different types of personalities to build your running business. It's free and you can pick and choose the areas of knowledge that best suit you.

chapter four

Salmon, grapes and a Moro bar

The weeks were whizzing by. I was up to ninety minutes' running and we were on target for the Woodbourne Half-marathon. Which was suddenly upon us. The Irishman dropped me and Gaz at the airport for the flight to Blenheim and wished us well. You'll be fine, love, he said. See you on Monday. And off he went. We were staying at a fabulous resort, the Vintner's Retreat, and it was fab — just like Wisteria Lane. I rattled around my three-bedroom townhouse like a truly desperate housewife and thanked the running gods and the resort owners for the fabulous spa bath in the high-tech bathroom. That would come in handy after the half. We enjoyed a quiet meal in the hotel restaurant and retired to our respective beds. I read for a while, told myself everything would be fine and slept like a log.

The morning, however, was a different prospect. My stomach was churning, but on my trainer's advice, I choked down some breakfast. It was a chilly Marlborough morning but I barely noticed the cold, I was so nervous. The plan was for Gaz to run the first 10 km with me, and then I was on my own. Having sustained some fair old injuries himself during his triathlon days, Gaz was only just coming back into training and he wanted to take it easy. We got to the start line bright and early and stood around shuffling and chatting nervously. 'We should warm up,' said Gaz. Just a gentle jog to the end of the sports field and back. About five paces in, I got the stitch. 'I can't even run four hundred metres,' I gasped. 'I can't do this.' 'Course you can,' said Gaz, the seasoned competitor. 'It's just nerves.'

There were about two hundred people taking part in the half — walkers and runners — and as is usual, the walkers headed off first. The day was warming up and turning into one of those beautiful, clear-blue Marlborough days. The route took us through vineyards, across farmland and onto the open road before returning to base and it was fairly flat and uncomplicated. We assembled at the start line and then we were off. The rest of the crowd shot off like hares and there was soon a considerable gap between me, Gaz and the rest of the pack. 'We're going to be last,' I wailed in between gasps.

When you're used to running at your own pace, it's disconcerting and off-putting to have to run at a pace set by other people. And to be passed by people you would naturally assume would be lower down the fitness scale than you. Like people fifteen years older. And 10 kilos heavier. And with physical afflictions. And especially, as happened ten minutes into the Woodbourne Half, by older, fatter men with heavily strapped knees who ran like bowlegged cowboys. How in God's name could somebody like that run past me? It was insulting. It was insensitive.

There must have been a bylaw somewhere that prohibited old, overweight pensioners with gimpy knees from running past women trying to better themselves. I felt like turning around, jogging back to the main road and thumbing a lift with any motorist who would take me to the nearest vineyard. I was seriously considering it, but my trainer knew me well by now and could sense trouble.

'Isn't it funny,' he said conversationally, 'how people take off at the start? It's not a sprint, it's a marathon. Pretty stupid, really. Still, it will be fun picking them off later in the race.'

'Yes,' I said, perking up immediately. 'It will. I'm not slow, really, am I? We're just conserving energy.'

'That's right,' said Gaz. 'You'll be fine. Just enjoy it.'

And within a few ks, I got into my own rhythm. I found that I was catching up with some of the other runners and settling into my own pace.

It was a truly gorgeous day but getting hotter with every passing minute. We hit the 10 km mark at a farmhouse and I gulped down the water on offer gratefully. This was the point at which Gaz was supposed to turn back, but he decided he'd carry on. He was feeling good and, besides, we were at the midway point with no obvious way of getting back, other than on foot. He was going to stay with me to the end. I wanted to kiss him, but I needed every last breath of air. Up over the hill, down the other side and onto the open road.

We were joined by a freckle-faced kid on a bike who informed us cheerfully that we had 'ages' to go. He was acting as support crew for his dad I think, and although my spirits had plummeted when he pointed out how far we still had to run, I cheered up considerably when he told us his dad was miles behind us. Gaz asked him what he had in his bag and the kid said he had a couple of Moro bars and would we like one? Would we? We almost mugged the little guy. He said he'd ride on ahead and have the Moro bar ready for us so we wouldn't have to stop, and off he pedalled. Sure enough, a couple of hundred metres ahead, there he was with a recently denuded Moro bar held out at the ready. Gaz broke it in two and we shared it between us. I swear that Moro bar was one of the best things I've ever tasted. They're quite chewy things, but where there's a will, there's a way and I managed to breathe, masticate and run, a superb example of multi-tasking. The sugar surged through me and gave me a new lease of life and there we were at the 16 km mark — just 5 km to go.

The sweat was pouring off us. The Marlborough grapes of 2006 should prove an interesting vintage, what with my sweat and the pee from the male runners who kept leaping off the road and into the vineyards. By now the cheerful chat between Gaz and me had pretty much dried up, but we enjoyed the encouragement of our wee friend on the bike. There were very few spectators — in fact, from memory there were none — so we had to supply our own motivation. The final drinks stop was at 19 km and I gulped down more water. There was the dearest little Border collie puppy under the drinks table and I couldn't resist stopping to pat him. Come on, said Gaz. We could come in under two hours if we get a move on. I couldn't have given a fat rat's bum. The fact that I was still alive I considered a minor miracle and *finishing* was the goal, not finishing in under two hours.

I felt dreadful that I was holding my fit young trainer back, but he shouldn't even have been running. I was saving him from his own testosterone by faffing around with the pup. Off we set for the final 2 km, and there it was. The finish line. We crossed over the line, shared a sweaty embrace and checked our times. Two hours and three minutes. If I hadn't stopped to pat the puppy, we would indeed have gone under two. But it didn't matter. I had completed a half-marathon, I was still alive and I was halfway to my goal of running a marathon. It was a real feeling of accomplishment. I enjoyed the text messages of support from my friends and family and it really does mean something when people take the time to let you know they're thinking of you. And as for my trainer . . . imagine being able to run a half-marathon on the spur of the moment. There's a lot to be said for being a fit young god with zero per cent body fat. Our relationship had evolved from a prickly first meeting to one of genuine trust and respect. I cannot speak too highly of the man — I'd even managed to get my head around calling him Gaz. For about two months I called him darling or umm — but one day, Gaz fell out of my mouth and Gaz he has been ever since.

We saw our little mate with the Moro bar at the prize-giving. I called him over and gave him ten bucks, thanked him for his kindness and told him to shout himself a treat. He was a well brought up wee lad and refused the money, but I insisted and he finally pocketed the dosh and we parted, both well pleased with our encounter.

We enjoyed a magnificent spa bath back at the hotel, each in our own individual baths, I hasten to add. All relationships with trainers are close, but if you're serious about your training, I don't think the relationship should ever be one of corporeal closeness. If all you want is a hottie to parade in front of your friends, then go for it, but I needed to run a marathon and I was only interested in Gaz's talent as a trainer. And I know he would have rather eaten his bike shorts than entertained this old girl in any carnal sense. I'm not being prurient in mentioning this: I've known some people to fall head over heels in love with their trainers with disastrous consequences. They're holding your leg above their head, your groin, thinly covered in Lycra is pressed right up against their thigh, they're staring into your eyes and you're talking about you — sounds like the basis for an excellent relationship. But when you're paying somebody by the hour, it is not an equal or indeed a real relationship. Don't bonk your trainer — it's a simple rule to live by.

I digress. We headed off for lunch and afterwards we rewarded ourselves with a mini wine trail. The lunch tasted great and although we were a bit stiff after sitting at the café for an hour, we soon warmed up after several wine tastings at the beautiful Marlborough wineries. I bought a bottle of Wither Hills pinot to enjoy after the Auckland Marathon and Gaz wrote out a training programme for one of the girls at Cloudy Bay who wanted to run a triathlon. We celebrated with a magnificent dinner and a few more wines back at our hotel. There's nothing like earning your food and I certainly felt that I had done so that day.

We both pulled up OK after the run. We checked out of our hotel and headed off to Picton where we were to meet our sponsors, Regal Salmon, and stride the boundaries of their empire. They were very nice people and the salmon fishery was a slick operation. I liked thinking that the salmon that ended up on my plate spent its days in such gorgeous surroundings before being gently released from this world to the next. They had a process of killing the fish called Aquaessence, where the fish swam into a chamber and carbon dioxide was released into the water in such quantities that the fish went to sleep and then died. Would that my death be as peaceful as that of a well-bred salmon's. Gaz and I thanked the team at Regal Salmon for their support and then it was time for the flight to Auckland. We had a few days off training, and then we were back into it with a vengeance.

For some people, the completion of their first half-marathon can feel like the end. The build-up towards the race is intense and afterwards they find it hard to get back into training for the full marathon. They find it difficult to stay motivated and some even give up the goal of running 42 km. I was lucky that I never hit that wall. I knew after Woodbourne that the job was only halfway done. Regal Salmon were giving $5000 to the Cystic Fibrosis Association if I completed the Auckland Marathon. That was my task and while it was gratifying to have run Woodbourne, I would only consider my goal achieved once I'd crossed the finish line in Auckland.

Where I did nearly come undone was when my race photo from Woodbourne arrived in the mail. I was completely unprepared for what I saw. I looked absolutely horrendous and as though at any moment I was about to expire. Eyes rolling in my head, face contorted in pain, my great fat stomach hanging over my leggings — I looked like a white rhino that had just been shot in the arse by hunters. It was so hideous I almost gave up then and there. A person like me had no business running marathons. I was too fat to run them. Nobody else who ran looked like me. I looked like I should have been propping the Buller scrum, not scampering across Marlborough farmland. Even my normally supportive family weren't much help. After showing them the photo, there was a shocked and appalled silence.

'Oh dear God,' said Kate. 'Oh, Mum, that's terrible.'

The Irishman shot a nervous sideways glance at me and cleared his throat tentatively. 'Umm — perhaps it's those tight legging things? They don't look the best for running.'

The women from the Titirangi Tunnel Rats were sympathetic when I poured out my tale of woe to them the following Saturday morning. They told me that nobody — except perhaps Allison Roe, we all conceded — looks good running. In the olden days when photos were laid out on the tables for purchase in the hours following the marathon, people would buy the images of themselves to ensure nobody else got to see them and then they'd tear them up immediately. Other marathon organisers, like Woodbourne's, used to send out photos automatically and the women told me that when a suspicious-looking A4-sized envelope turned up in the mail in the weeks following an event, they'd just pop it straight in the rubbish without opening it. Sound advice and advice I wish I'd received before my Woodbourne photo arrived in my mailbox. It was a bad few days, but once I'd stuffed the photo at the bottom of the drawer and had a couple of days off, I'd put the incident behind me and was ready to tackle the final couple of months of my training.

GAZ

Without Kerre knowing, the half-marathon in Woodbourne was by far my most nerve-racking time of the training. This was when everybody was going to see if she had actually been training — and if the training plan, large support team and hype would pay off. Before the half a lot of people doubted that Kerre would do the training, let alone finish a marathon. Being the new kid on the block, I had something to prove as well. Although Kerre was happy that I decided to continue once we reached halfway, to be honest with you, I had no choice! I had to guard my investment — Kerre was similar to a sub-prime mortgage (high risk, high return!) and I wasn't about to let my eye off her. And besides, there were too many wineries open along the way and Kerre has a voracious appetite for wine. Someone had to keep her in check.

When we came across the finish line I felt a sense of relief and accomplishment, but that was very quickly followed by the realisation that I was knackered. I wish I had been able to put in a little training for the event. I covered up the fact that it hurt pretty well, I think!

Once Kerre had completed the half-marathon, things changed. People became increasingly interested in her journey and started to believe that she was going to run the marathon. Of course, this didn't bother us, but it was nice to know nonetheless.

Whether you're an amateur just starting out or an élite athlete training at the top of your game, sooner or later you will come across people who doubt you and don't want to see you succeed. Just remember that once you succeed, they will want to join the wagon. And that's OK; everyone is travelling their own journey.

It must be noted that Kerre set a fantastic time for her first half, 2:03:00. She followed her training programme to the letter, almost scarily, as I allow for sessions to be missed because I'm aware that everyone isn't perfect. She blew me away with her dedication to the cause and it paid off.

Completing your first half-marathon is a crucial part of marathon training. From this race you can determine how well your training has gone and you can roughly calculate your expected time for the marathon. The general rule of thumb is to multiply the half-marathon time by two and add twenty or thirty minutes. It's a little rough, but more times than not has proven accurate. It will only work, though, if you continue to train after you've run the half!

One last important training tip for the half: you need to run at least 18 km before the race. This will ensure that you get across the finish line safely and allows the body to adapt in a slow, progressive manner without overtraining. In saying that, don't be surprised if at the 17 km mark you feel like you've hit a small brick wall. Just hang in there, as this is all part of the build-up and is instrumental for your success in the big race. And besides, it's character building and gives you an insight into your personal mental and physical barriers.

chapter five

Pure indulgence

The hours were climbing up and I was running between 50 and 60 km a week, but I wasn't losing any weight. I imagined when I started this whole marathon-training business that I would eventually become an object of concern among my friends. 'She's lost so much weight,' they'd whisper to one another. 'Do you think she's overdoing the training? Should we say something?' I was mentally totting up how much it would cost to replace my entire wardrobe and, indeed, how much it would cost me in lost speaking opportunities if I became a shadow of my former self. Along with the radio, I also work as an MC and after-dinner speaker and a big part of my arsenal is my chest. Actually, the biggest part of my arsenal is my arse, but my chest is what they see first. When it's just you standing in front of six to seven hundred A-type personalities, all leaders and winners in their field, and it's just one 1.6-metre woman out there on the stage making them sit still and keep quiet, you need all the help you can get. And my boobs, trussed up and thrusting forwards, help to get their attention. I imagined as I faded away to a shadow of my former self that the tits and teeth work would dry up as well. Hah! Although I'd lost a few kilos, I was still sitting on 69 kilos — about 9 kilos heavier than I thought I'd be.

Gaz didn't want to know. 'I'm here to train you to run a marathon, not to help you lose weight. Go and talk to a nutritionist.' And so I did, and although she was lovely and a very good advertisement for the six small meals a day she advised, there was no way I was going to follow her advice. She told me the protein part of my meals should be able to fit into the palm of my hand — I'm sure you've heard this advice before. What a crock! I lasted a day doing my handfuls, and then I got the Irishman to hold out his hand while I spooned in the chicken and the rice and the veges — and when that wasn't enough either, I got him to cup both hands, which was a whole lot more satisfactory. Six small handfuls of food a day! Surely the advantage of running so many miles was that I could eat whatever the hell I liked and as much as I liked. And on those long Saturday morning runs, the thought of the hot bath the Irishman would have ready and the smoked salmon and cream cheese bagel that would follow was what got me through the last boring 5 km along the pipeline track. As my tired, sore feet carried me back towards Titirangi Village I fantasised about that bagel and the reality was every bit as good as the fantasy. Don't run a marathon if you want to lose weight. You will certainly change shape — I went down a dress size — and you will lose a few excess kilos but you won't become the sylphlike creature you imagine will be the payoff for running for fricking hours unless you do all the other boring things involved in dropping kilos — like cutting down on what you eat. And that's no fun.

Although I wasn't losing weight, my boobs were getting smaller. Just after I'd committed myself to running a marathon, I was phoned and told I was one of the winners of the Fayreform Best Breasts competition. Along with Charlotte Dawson, Nicky Watson, Rachel Hunter and Jacqui Brown among others, I was named as having one of the best racks in the country. It seemed a tad unfair to have my saggy breast-feeding boobs judged alongside Nicky and Charlotte's plastic fantastics — a bit like amateurs having to front up alongside professionals. To be honest, I think those who were chosen were selected partly for their ability to provide free publicity to Fayreform, rather than for the marvellousness of their mammaries, but hey! I'll take any award going. I think that makes me, technically, an award-winning journalist. Does anyone ever ask what award the award-winning journalist has won? No. Exactly. I have won an award; I am a journalist; ergo, I'm an award-winning journalist. QED. The prize was $500 worth of free lingerie from Bendon and although the other girls were rifling through the stands like truffle hunters on the scent, I told the lovely Bendon ladies I'd be back after I'd run the marathon. I thought that I'd probably change a bit by the time the marathon had been raced and I was right. I went from a 14DD to a 12C — even though I'd only lost a couple of kilos. I didn't have to give back the prize — and indeed, nor should I have had to. Within a couple of months of not running, I was back to my buxom best.

It was around about this time that I felt game enough to start wearing the gear that Regal Salmon had sent me. It was lovely stuff — adidas shirt, shorts, long-sleeved running jacket and track pants all branded up beautifully with their logos. I had put the whole lot in my bottom drawer when it first arrived as I had only just started running and didn't think I'd be a terribly flash advertisement for their product if I was heaving my way round the block, with my cheeks pinker than their finest salmon, looking like I was about to have a cardiac infarction at any moment. But after a couple of months of running, I felt confident that while the company probably wouldn't garner any sales as a result of my running round the street with their logo bouncing energetically on my chest, they shouldn't lose any custom either. So I opened the drawer and undid the parcel. And it was only then that I noticed the running shorts. They weren't branded with the logo — they were branded with the company slogan. So when I put on the shorts, there, stretched tight across my arse, were the words 'Pure Indulgence'. It looked like a government health warning. Twenty years of purely indulgent living and you too could have an arse like this! It was great. When I get back into racehorse syndicates, I want a big-bummed horse that I can call Pure Indulgence.

The last couple of months before a marathon is always danger time. The mileage builds up to a climax before you taper off and if anything's going to blow, the last six weeks will be the time it happens. It's also the time your mind starts playing tricks on you. You lie awake at night, staring at the ceiling like a possum in the headlights thinking, 'I haven't done enough. I'm too old/fat/unfit/unprepared — whatever — to run a marathon. What was I thinking?' On and on it goes. Boring as buggery, but there's precious little you can do about it. I recommend getting pissed.

I was due to do a long run with Bruce and the girls one Saturday morning, but I had to attend a fundraiser the night before. It was a Plunket fundraiser, so I couldn't not go — besides, I wanted to. Norm Hewitt and Shane Cortese and Lorraine Mexted and Beatrice Faumuina were going to be there, dancing, and I loved *Dancing with the Stars*. Mel, one of the producers of *Intrepid Journeys*, was going to be my date, as the Irishman never goes anywhere and Mel and I were both in the mood for a bit of a play. Play we did and I ended up rolling home from the Hyatt at two in the morning after drinking, officially, two and off the record, five, stonking great glasses of red wine. When the alarm went off at six the next morning, I was not a happy camper. I felt ill and disoriented from a combination of lack of sleep and yes, OK, booze.

I was supposed to be meeting Lee and driving her to the run. If I'd had her number I would have phoned her and told her I was sick. But I didn't and I couldn't bear the thought of her waiting in the cool morning air for the ride that never came. So I crawled out of bed, dragged on my gear and headed round the corner to pick her up. Before I could start on my litany of woes, Lee got in first. She was exhausted from lack of sleep and overwork and only the thought of me coming to pick her up got her out of bed. We bitched and moaned our way down to the waterfront where we were to meet Lavina and Bruce, our running guru.

I mentioned Bruce earlier and it's now time to properly introduce him. We four were so lucky to have him take an interest in our running. A young and fit-looking sixty, Bruce Matthews joined the Titirangi Tunnel Rats when he and his family immigrated to New Zealand in 1994. While he was living in South Africa, he earned the right to a permanent number in the Comrades Marathon — the punishing 90 km run that alternates annually between the uphill run from Durban to Pietermaritzburg and the downhill version of the same track, Pietermaritzburg to Durban. Bruce has run it twenty times. He also trained a young woman to victory in the Comrades and in the course of running more than 150 marathons, he's gone under 2:30 more than ten times. In his fourteen years in New Zealand, he's also earned the right to a permanent number in the adidas Auckland Marathon — we were in the company of greatness.

And now he'd made it his personal mission to ensure Lee, Lavina, Mary and I were in the best shape possible to run our marathons. Why? I know, I asked the same thing. Why would an élite athlete who was used to working with the best get up early on a Saturday morning to plod along with a middle-aged back of the packer (I speak of myself only here — the other girls were in far better nick than me). When I asked him, he grinned and told me it was all about giving back. He'd had a ball, and he'd been helped along the way, and he wanted us to experience the joy of running a marathon. We couldn't quite believe our luck in having Bruce on our side, but not wanting to look a gift marathoner in the mouth, we accepted any suggestions gratefully and acquiesced to his ideas.

That morning the plan was to run along Auckland's waterfront — a good 20 km run — and test our different energy gels to use during our respective marathons. I didn't think I could walk from the car park to the waterfront. But we did, and Bruce and Lavina turned up minutes later.

Off we went. Lavina and Lee shot off and Bruce stayed behind with me, bless him. The motion of the running was making me feel ill and I was so tired I think I nodded off a couple of times while we ran. Five km later we stopped for a drink of water at the fountain, and Bruce suggested we try one of the running gels. That almost finished me off completely. Imagine a bodily emission — any one, they're all equally gross — heavily laced with sucrose and fruit flavouring. It was like swallowing a big cup of warm, sweet snot. I almost barfed. I spat it out immediately and stuck with the water. We set off again and then we were at the turnaround. Ten km down, ten to go. The sun was out now and so were the beautiful people heading off for their Saturday morning brunches at the trendy seafront cafés. I hated them all. But it was one foot in front of the other and Bruce telling me stories of past marathon glories and as the alcohol left my body and the endorphins kicked in, I truly began to feel better. And two hours later it was over. 'You'll be fine,' said Lavina. 'You've just run a half-marathon without wanting to be here.' She was right. From that moment on, I knew I would make it, because no matter how bad I was feeling on the day of the marathon itself, there was absolutely no way I could possibly feel worse than I did that day.

It was shortly after that run, though, that I felt a hamstring twinge. And I panicked. I was so far through my training and the marathon was so close that the only thing worse than running the marathon would be *not* being able to run the bloody thing. Whether it was the Waitakere hills or the speed work Gaz introduced, whatever, there was a twinge. Just to be on the safe side, I gave running a rest for a while and took to the pool. Emile was my aqua-jogging trainer — a man who'd run a couple of marathons himself — so he knew his stuff. And so down to the Tepid Pools I went to don a flotation belt and wrist and ankle weights and jog up and down the pool. For hours. Even with Emile's company, it was mind-numbingly dull. But needs must. And I'd read enough on the coolrunning.com website to know that aqua-jogging is an acceptable substitute if injury prevents you from taking to the roads.

Emile brought my entourage to eight. Eight people I had consulted to get me through my marathon mission. I saw Gaz at least a couple of times a week. Kiri was my masseuse and she was invaluable. I had been used to the sort of massages you get from beauty therapists — you know, beautiful soft-voiced girls with names like Isabella or Tiffany who tell you in whispers that they're about to use the ylang ylang oil now and who rub your back in a most soothing and comforting way. Although she was beautiful and soft voiced, there was nothing bloody soothing about Kiri's massages. I bellowed like a bull calf who'd just become a steer the first time Kiri massaged me. And although my pain tolerance built up quickly, there is nothing comfortable about having your quads or your IT band massaged. It's necessary, but it's not nice.

Then there was Iain, one of the first professionals other than Gaz I consulted. He saw me every couple of weeks to click me back into shape. It made sense. If your body's out of alignment then the continual pounding of running is going to further compound the injury. So every second Friday I'd present myself at the chiropractor's, where the suave former rugby player would lay me out on the table, flip me round a bit, then boot me out the door. Reminded me of my skanky old waitress days in the eighties. Actually, he's become a vital part of my family's ongoing health and he's fixed a couple of aches and pains that I'd been carrying for nearly twenty years. I don't think I could have made it without him.

Also on my team were Fiona the nutritionist, James the podiatrist, James the orthopaedic surgeon, Tim the physio and the aforementioned Emile, the aqua-jogging coach. Some of them I saw only once or twice but still, it was costing me a bloody fortune, even with Regal Salmon paying for Gaz. However, if a job's worth doing, it's worth doing right. I wasn't smoking and I've never done drugs — except alcohol, and even that I'd cut back on a bit. Besides, I was committed to getting though the marathon without crippling myself. It was a massive investment of time and a considerable amount of money, but I was lucky that I could afford both to achieve my goal. On good weeks, I was spending less than $100 a week; bad ones, up to $200. If you are going to run a marathon you don't have to spend as much as I did. I know some people who spent more and plenty who spent less. But at some stage you will need to consult health professionals and it might pay to keep an emergency stash set aside just in case you need to go to see a podiatrist or get X-rays done.

One of the main things stressed in marathon training regimes is the importance of doing the long run. As I've mentioned, the long run is generally done on the weekend, when you have time to do it and time to recover. As your training progresses, the long runs get longer, building to a climax of 30 to 35 km before you begin the equally important taper — the cutting down of kilometres run and the resting of the body before assaulting it with a marathon. My dodgy hammy meant my long, long run had to be put off and we were running out of time. The last weekend I could possibly do it was a weekend I was booked to MC the Tauranga Chamber of Commerce Business Awards and I was dreading the prospect of running the longest I'd ever run on my own and in a city I didn't know. I was absolutely delighted when Lavina said she would run with me, as she lived in Tauranga and would be at home that weekend, and even more delighted when Lee said she and her family would be visiting Lavina that weekend and she would come too. Mary Lambie had headed off to Iran on an *Intrepid Journey* where she was having to try to juggle New York Marathon training with filming commitments. Can you imagine trying to run in a burqa? Mary did and footage is available on DVD.

However, back to Tauranga. Lavina rang to say she and Lee would meet me outside my hotel at 7 a.m. and we would head off to Mount Maunganui, where we would run around the Mount and then jog back to Tauranga and my hotel. Lavina's dad, a former marathon runner who was visiting from Australia, had promised he would meet us along the way and bring water. Sounded like a plan, so I told the girls I'd see them in the morning and headed out to do my tits and teeth for Tauranga. It was a great night, as these events usually are, and there was a lovely dinner — and although I limited my wine consumption to just a couple of glasses, it was still 1 a.m. by the time I got back to the hotel. The owners had kindly given me a lift back, and as one of them had run the Comrades Marathon, they'd taken an interest in my training and had offered to provide me with what I needed for the run in the morning. I shall never forget the look on a lovely English couple's faces when, just as the lift doors were closing to take us three guests up to our room, the manager said, 'I'll have the Vaseline and the banana brought up to your room in just a few minutes.' The English couple's faces turned to stone and the air in the small lift turned frigid and I began to stammer out an explanation and then I just started laughing and that was the end of that.

The Vaseline and banana did indeed get delivered to my room, but I was exhausted after the drive from Auckland and the adrenalin from performing and slept through my alarm. The first thing I knew was the phone ringing and Lee asking me where the hell was I? I threw on my clothes, choked down the banana and headed down, full of apologies, to meet the girls. I don't know whether it was the rushed start or the new running route or whether I didn't have a back-of-the-packer to run with so went out too fast, but that run was a bastard. I hated every moment of it, apart from the beauty of running around the Mount. It was hot, it was hard and it was ugly. I had the stitch for most of the way, my foot hurt and I was metres behind the other two girls. But again, bailing out wasn't an option — besides, what could I do? I had no way to ring a cab, no money to pay for one, and there was no way in God's earth anyone would have picked me up if I'd decided to hitchhike — so it was one foot in front of the other and head for home. About a kilometre from the hotel, I spotted a familiar figure in the distance and sure enough as I got closer I saw it was Jonah Lomu out walking with one of his provincial rugby team-mates.

'Crikey!' he exclaimed. 'What are you doing?' I came to a grateful stop and told the girls to go on without me and I'd meet them back at the hotel. Well, it would have been rude not to talk to Jonah. He's lovely. And besides, he did look quite concerned.

I told him I'd been running to the Mount and back because I was training for a marathon. His young team-mate looked incredulous.

'Why?' he asked. I told him when he hit forty and had a midlife crisis, he would understand. Women have menopause. Men go through meno-Porsche when they trade in the old wife for a hot new young thing and exchange the family sedan for a fire engine-red Porsche. Same but different. So we all exchanged pleasantries for a couple of minutes and I set off again to cover the last kilometre. And that was it. My only really big run was about 6 to 10 km light. Although Gaz told me I'd done enough, every single training bible said the 32 km run was vitally important as a physical and psychological component to running a marathon. I'd peaked at 26. But it was too late to do anything about that. I'd run out of time to complete a longer run. Now all that was left for me to do was taper — and worry.

GAZ

Nutrition plays a very large role in running, though most people like running because they can eat what they want (Kerre included). It must be stressed that the food we put into our mouths fuels the engine that will move our legs at approximately 10,000 steps per hour when running. You wouldn't put diesel in a petrol engine and equally, if you were driving Formula One, you wouldn't fill your tank with too much fuel, as you want to be operating as light as possible. Running is no different. I always refer my clients to a nutritionist, as everyone is different and needs tailor-made food plans. I also encourage clients to educate themselves and learn the basics of carbohydrates, fats and proteins, and the importance of each. A great read on nutrition is *Optimum Sports Nutrition* by Dr Michael Colgan.

It may intrigue you to know that runners work through as much protein as a bodybuilder, and we all know how much those overzealous, protein-loading, iron-pushing folk consume! Breakdown and repair of proteins is a part of the natural life cycle of muscle tissue and it is exacerbated by increased physical activity. We must replace those proteins through our dietary intake, whether in food or supplements.

I would love to say that running is a very safe sport, but the reality is that approximately 90 per cent of runners experience some sort of injury at some time. Each strike of each leg carries the full weight of the body behind it. If the runner does not take sufficient time to allow their body to adapt to this stress, and if they don't adopt a proactive approach to injury prevention, the risk of injury increases greatly. Ninety per cent of the injured runners I see have run too much, too soon and lack sufficient overall body strength to cope with the speed at which they are running. If you are going to start running, make sure the programme intensity is right and follow these simple rules:

- Train frequently and consistently.
- Start gradually and train gently.
- Train first for distance, then later for speed.

A first-year runner should never tackle intervals or specific hill work. During that first year your whole focus should be on adapting your body to the stress of running.

You have to be proactive about injury prevention. Consult a professional who can help to identify any potential problems that may arise once you start running. They will be able to tell you what to look out for and, more importantly, how to deal with any injuries that arise. The body gives out 100 signs before it actually succumbs to injury. By listening to your body you can often prevent an injury occurring. Even if you do end up with an injury, try to turn it into a positive experience. Learn from it — once you have been through an injury and come out the other side, you will be much more informed about the human body and its healthy function. The ability to read the signals from your own body is priceless, not just for sport but for general health as well.

As a running specialist, I offer an initial consultation to determine whether or not a person has the base strength and structural stability that is needed for running. If a person does not have enough core strength, or their muscle or skeletal system is unbalanced, then that will make things difficult for them when they run. For instance, a weak left hip would likely cause stress in the right leg, resulting in a tightening of the iliotibial band (a tendon that runs from the hip and inserts into the knee), and this could cause knee tendonitis. This is an extreme example, but if it was left uncorrected, it would stop you running. If you have problems like this, though, it's not the end of the world. It just means you might have to spend six months working out in the gym and walking to prepare your body for running.

When you are training for a distance run, a good sports

massage is essential. It can often help you avoid injury. It's a great idea to find a practitioner who deals with runners on a regular basis. Generally speaking, all runners follow a similar pattern of tightness and injury and a specific running masseur will be aware of this.

If you are training for a half-marathon, then one massage per fortnight is sufficient. Once you step up your training for a marathon, increase your massage frequency to once a week. If you ignore tight and sore muscles they will end up costing you precious training time and, worse, may result in injury.

Regular sports massage is just one of the costs involved in any running programme. Never underestimate the cost of maintaining your running habit. If you are going to run in a safe and effective manner and want to enjoy the champagne once you've crossed the finish line, then take some of these costs into consideration:

- Running programme/running assessment and running-specific strength programme: $340–$400
- Ongoing monthly programme and strength programme progression: $80–$100
- Further strength sessions: $80–$100 (per one-on-one session), $30–$40 (per group session). Two sessions a week are recommended.
- Specialist consultant (if an injury arises or for preventative assessments): $90–$140 initially and $45–$90 for subsequent consultations
- Massage: $70–$90 per session
- Shoes: $300–$380 per pair (average wear is two pairs up to the marathon)

- Clothes: $170–$200 per set (shorts, top, socks, sports bra, underwear).

Kerre was spending up to $200 a week on a bad week. If you're on a tight budget then at least allow $70 a week. Do not start training for a marathon unless you are aware of the costs involved and able to meet them from your disposable income. Something as seemingly minor as not renewing your shoes on time or leaving your massage a week too long could be the difference between an injury and good running health.

chapter six

The first final hurdle

And worry I did. For about two weeks before the marathon, I panicked. I don't know how international sportsmen cope with the pressure. All I had to do was stagger around 42 km, collapse over the line, and finish. Nobody cared what time I ran the race in, and certainly nobody expected me to even come close to winning it. All I had to do was finish. And I could do that even if I crawled. But your mind plays tricks on you. I thought of all the people who'd put their time and expertise and energy into seeing me to the start line. They'd done their bit — what if I couldn't do mine and I failed to finish? Imagine how let down they'd feel! And what about the lovely people from the Cystic Fibrosis Association? What if I failed them a second time? What if I folded like I'd folded at the charity poker tournament? On and on, and around and around it went. I was pretty much in a blue funk and it was getting worse as the day got closer.

One of the worst days was when I was hosting a function for Caltex and their retailers at Sky City's Sky Tower. We'd had a lovely dinner and I'd done my bit and one of the service station owners asked me where exactly I'd be running in a fortnight. Standing at the top of the Sky Tower, with its gorgeous panoramic view, it was easy to map out the route.

Well, I said, pointing out to the left, we start at Devonport and then we run to Takapuna, then it's up to Northcote, across the Harbour Bridge and along the waterfront . . . My voice started to trail off as I stared at the route I would have to run. It was a phenomenal distance. What was I thinking? There was no way I could run 42 km! I broke out in a cold sweat and smiled wanly when the lovely Caltex crowd told me they'd be thinking of me and wasn't it a tremendous effort? Some experts suggest you drive the route of the marathon you're about to run so you can visualise it in your mind, work out strategies for the hills — things like that. I don't know. Visualising it didn't work for me. I almost pulled out that night.

As part of the hosting for Caltex, I had to MC their final awards dinner. It was to be held in the Town Hall and was black tie and terribly grand. I'd been working with them during the day, then tore up the hill to the lovely team at Servilles in Ponsonby, who do the sow's ear/silk purse routine for me most weekends. As usual, I only had an hour for Aneez, my stylist, to work his magic, and, as usual, I'd be changing in the Servilles loos before charging back down the hill to the Town Hall for rehearsals and sound check.

Gone are the days when a girl could drag a comb through her hair, put on a clean frock and a bit of lippy and just turn up. Bloody Charlotte Dawson's got a lot to answer for! When that glamour girl turned up from Oz and started doing the rounds of the speaking circuit, all the other girls had to lift their game. Now, before I even get to the event, I've spent the better part of half a day getting a spray tan, a manicure, my hair styled and my make-up done, complete with false lashes and artful shading. The team and I have it down to a fine art now. My dress, shoes and jewellery were in the car and the moment I was done, one of the lovely girls offered to go out to the car and grab my dress and the other bits and pieces.

'I'll just need the car keys,' she said.

Right. The car keys. My phone was there but there were no car keys lying next to the phone. They weren't at reception. They weren't at the desk, and they weren't in my handbag, because I very seldom carry a handbag. Another organisational flaw in my life. The entire salon was tipped upside down, other clients were checking their handbags — it was chaos. I didn't have time to get home for another dress and, besides, I didn't have the key to get into the house. Aneez, my stylist, suddenly snapped his fingers.

'Sit down, stop panicking — you'll ruin the make-up — and have a glass of water,' he said, and disappeared out the door. Within ten minutes, he was back, a gorgeous golden gown over one arm and a pair of strappy gold stilettos dangling from one finger. He'd gone to the dress shop down the road and found an evening dress and taken it into the shoe shop next door and matched a pair of shoes for me. The retailers were happy to let me borrow these items for the night, thanks to Aneez, and it looked like Cinderella would be going to the ball after all. I tried the outfit on in the loos and it was damn near perfect. The cross-over top gaped a bit as I didn't have the right strap-em-up-and-push-em-out bra on, and the gown was too long, but otherwise I looked every inch the professional MC. Aneez shot across the road to a jewellery store and borrowed a brooch, which he used to pin the top, but even he couldn't fix the length of the dress.

'It won't matter,' I said. 'I'll be behind a podium — no-one will ever know.' And they say you pay too much to go to the hairdressers! Honestly, without the crew at Servilles, there's no way I would be able to keep the show on the road. This is just one example of what they can do.

I did, however, have to take off my shoes to walk down the very steep stairs that lead from the top of the Town Hall down to the stage. I had a long, long dress on and brand new slippery shoes — the last thing I needed two weeks before running a marathon was to trip and sprain an ankle. Like I say, the only thing worse than running the marathon would be not running it. So I glided down to the stage barefoot, and at the first break I shot backstage and popped off the shoes. I wasn't willing to take any chances!

The other bad moment was just two days before the marathon. You have to queue to get your race pack and when I saw the length of the queue snaking out from the race headquarters at the Viaduct, I had a meltdown. A combination of sheer terror and lack of sleep combined to make me pull out my mobile and shriek at lovely Antonia from Pead PR.

'There's a million people here and I haven't got time to queue and I can't do it anyway and this is just awful!' This was sort of the gist of what I was saying, although I have no doubt to Antonia it sounded like hysterical gibberish.

'There, there,' she said in her soothing, calm, unflappable way. 'It's going to be fine. Do you want me to come down and queue for you?' That brought me back to my senses. The thought of this busy, intelligent professional coming down and standing in a line for me to get my race pack because I was too pathetic to get it myself was like a bucket of cold water. I said that I would be fine, I'd do it myself and I was sorry to have bothered her.

The week before the marathon I received the most beautiful letter from Alex Powell, the Auckland president of the Cystic Fibrosis Association. I hadn't met her before — I'd just nominated the charity as the one that would receive the cheque and got on with the training — but Alex took the time to write to me and tell me how much it meant that I was undertaking the marathon for the association. Alex and her husband have three beautiful girls and the youngest, Isabella, has cystic fibrosis.

CF is New Zealand's most common inherited life-threatening disease, with one in 3000 babies diagnosed with it. The association says that living with CF is like running a marathon every day, given the problems these kids have with their lungs. It's a cruel disease as so many young people are able, through tremendous effort, to live relatively normal lives. They're bright, they play sport, but they're on a shortened time-line and it's made doubly cruel for the families who are given these beautiful kids to love — but only for a short time. The life expectancy for CF sufferers is getting longer, thanks to the advances that have been made in scientific research and medical treatment, but still, most kids diagnosed with CF are lucky to make it past thirty.

Alex included a photo of Bella, and to have a picture of the wee girl I'd be running for made the world of difference. It certainly put my training and effort into perspective and I was looking forward to meeting the girls in person. Alex was actually going to be running the Auckland Half, so I was keen to compare notes with her after the event.

As well as Alex's letter, I also received a heart-warming letter of encouragement from the team at Regal Salmon. The card was signed by all of the workers, some of whom Gaz and I had met when we were in Marlborough running the Woodbourne Half. A lot of my listeners on the radio had sent through emails and texts of support too, so I didn't feel alone. We were running a sweepstake on the radio — people had to guess how long it would take me to run the Auckland Marathon. A few optimistic souls put in times around the two-hour mark; one snide coot put in five days! But Gaz and I were working on five hours — fifteen minutes less if all went well.

I didn't want to aim for a time. My main goal was to finish and collapse into the arms of my family. I'd extracted a promise from the Irishman and my daughter that they would be there for me at the end. I needed to know that they would be there when I finished. Even though Kate had a big party on the Saturday night, she vowed she'd be at the finishing line. And I knew the Irishman would be. He had to compensate for a previous indiscretion when I'd walked the Tongariro Crossing for charity. That was a long, hard, four-hour hike and towards the end the only thing that kept me going was the thought of seeing my lovely man's beautiful face. But when I got to the end, he wasn't there. He wasn't in the massage room. He wasn't anywhere. Well, in fact, he was. He was asleep on the bed in our room at the Chateau, having knocked himself out watching telly. If my feet hadn't hurt so much, I'd have walked out on him. It was one of those crimes that partners hurl at one another decades after the transgression. I promised him that if he was at the finish of the Auckland Marathon, I would never, ever speak of the Horror of the Tongariro Crossing and his Subsequent Failure to Be at the Line ever again. He swore faithfully he would be there (and probably swore at me under his breath, too) so that was one less thing to worry about. I received a phone call from Iran, too. Mel was directing Mary in her *Intrepid Journey* just as she'd directed me in Cambodia and the two of them rang to wish me luck. Mary was flying to New York the day after she got back from Iran and she promised to email me her race number so I could follow her progress online. We were both full of trepidation but assured each other all would be well.

And then it was the day before. Months and months ago, before I'd even run the Woodbourne Half, I'd booked a room at the Esplanade Hotel in Devonport when I'd realised what time the marathon started. There was no way I was going to wake up at 4.30, catch a ferry and make it to the start line, let alone make it to the finish line. I simply couldn't imagine acheiving that level of organisation. So I rang and made a reservation at the hotel. After a lovely carbo-rich lunch of smoked salmon and pasta, the Irishman and I headed over to Devonport, took a leisurely walk around North Head with the dog, and then they deposited me at my digs for the night. I had everything I needed for the night and the marathon and we were going to come back after the run to pick up my gear. I'd been drinking sports drink throughout the day and for dinner I nibbled on nuts and fruit. I had a couple of good books and I set my alarm for 5.45 a.m. — the very latest I could possibly leave it. The race started outside the door of the hotel so I only had to roll out of bed, ready myself and walk down the stairs of the pub. There was nothing more that I could do. The training was over and D-day was less than twelve hours away. I slept fitfully, but then I hadn't had a good night's sleep in weeks. And as I lay there lying in the bed staring at the ceiling like a possum in the headlights the alarm went off. Today was the day I was going to become a marathon runner — or die trying.

From the moment I got up, I felt great. It was a beautiful morning, clear and still, and the nervous energy running through the crowd of runners and walkers was stimulating. Amongst the crowd, I found Tim, the *Herald* editor, and his friends, and we resolved to run the first few ks together. We all jostled together nervously and waited for the gun to go off. And on the dot of 6.30 it did, but given the numbers of people, it took a few minutes before we actually crossed the start line. I felt great — no aches, no pains, no stitch and Tim and I chatted away until we got to Northcote, where he lengthened his stride and peeled away. I pootled along enjoying the scenery and taking my time, but I felt a real excitement when we ran onto the motorway and headed towards the Harbour Bridge. It was great being able to run on the bridge and I shouted myself one of my jelly dinosaurs that I was keeping in my back pocket for energy. The baby jelly dinosaurs had morphed into one great *Tyrannosaurus rex*, what with the combination of my body heat and the jiggling of my butt, but what the heck. I just bit his head off, enjoyed the sugar kick and revelled in the experience.

We came off the bridge and headed round through the Tank Farm and that's where I saw the first of the bodies. Up until that point, I hadn't seen any walking wounded, no ambulances, no sign that anything was amiss. But with about 1 km to go to the end of the half-marathon, people were dropping like flies. I think I passed about six of them, men and women, mainly youngies, either passed out or collapsed on the side of the road, unable to go another step. It seemed such a shame. There was such a wee way to go, but I guess when you get to that state, another step would seem monumental, another kilometre impossible to contemplate. There were people lining the streets, urging on the half-marathoners — come on, not long now, you're almost there! I knew I was only halfway there, but at no time did I feel resentful of those who would be enjoying the congratulations and the cold drinks and the massages within minutes. I'd come to run a marathon and I had another couple of hours to go.

Gaz rode by on his bike and asked me how I was feeling. We chatted and I told him the only problem was not being able to open the tube of Peak Fuel sucrose paste. I'd been munching on dinosaurs, but for the final 21 km I probably needed something a bit more scientific. He grabbed the tube as I jogged along next to him and used the cap to pierce the seal. Not so hard after all, really. He wished me well and told me he'd see me at the finish. It was good to see a friendly face. Tim the physio lived in an apartment in the Viaduct and he was on the side of the road too, to cheer along his clients. And then there was Bruce — cooling his heels, waiting for me to turn up. He had seen his wife through the half-marathon and, as he'd promised, he would run with me for the last half of the marathon. He told me I was looking fit and fresh and, without wishing to sound like John Mitchell, we set off for the second half of the journey.

The run along the waterfront was tough. It was a straight out and back — out to St Heliers then back to Victoria Park for the finish. I'd run it before and I knew what I was in for. It's long and flat and boring and the lovely clear morning had turned into an overcast, windy day. There were few spectators along the route, so I was delighted to see my mate Jane standing at the 26 km mark. Jane is the other half of the team that produces *Intrepid Journeys*, and she was the one who'd had the misfortune to see my G-string blister. Normally, she would be in some far-off exotic location making television, but having a baby had clipped her wings for a minute or two. She'd been a keen runner in her day and there she was, with a bag of bananas in one hand and a steak and cheese pie in the other. 'I didn't want to miss you,' she called out as I jogged towards her, 'so I grabbed breakfast on the way.' I gave her a sweaty hug, scoffed down half a banana, and then set off again.

'I'll run a wee way with you,' she said. And she did. And the faces of the people along the route were priceless as they saw a tiny wee woman with the biggest breasts in the southern hemisphere — they were impressive before she started breastfeeding — running in the Auckland Marathon while eating a steak and cheese pie. The shaming thing is she managed to keep pace with me for a few ks before she dropped off and told me she'd see me on her way home.

The morale boost you get from a friendly face — and indeed, a magnificent set of tits — is remarkable. If you know you have someone waiting for you at a designated point, it gives you something to look forward to, it takes your mind off yourself and alleviates the boredom. Your head comes up, your pace quickens, and two or three ks have gone by without you noticing. It's brilliant. The best thing is to con some sucker into running the marathon with you. The next best thing is to gather together a support crew. If you have friends, beg or bribe them to stand for hours on a chilly street just to yell encouragement for a couple of minutes as you go by. If you don't have friends, find some before you run your marathon. I am very, very grateful to those hardy souls who did come down to cheer me on. You'll all be remembered in my will.

We hit the turnaround at St Heliers and then we were on the homeward straight. Still more than 11 km to go, but hey, what's 11 km when you've just run 30? With about 6 or 7 km to go, though, I was starting to fade. I wasn't tired so much as losing interest. Bored. I'd been running for more than three hours, and although nothing hurt, nothing ached, I was bored. Bruce had a plan. 'See those guys up ahead,' he said. 'Pick up the pace and we can take them.'

'I don't want to,' I whined. 'I'm OK — it's not about my time; it's just finishing.'

'Come on,' he said, 'you're getting lazy. Let's pick out people and pass them.' With that, he lengthened his stride and I had the choice of losing my running mate or going with him. The boys up ahead looked young and strong —

and they also looked completely and utterly shagged. They had obviously gone out to run the mother of all marathons. They were going to rewrite the history books and they weren't going to stop for water because that was just for pussies — and now they'd hit the wall and they were doing it hard over the last 6 km. Bruce and I overtook the young bucks. 'Not long to go,' I called out cheerily as we jogged on ahead of them. Behind me I heard a groan that came deep from the soul of one of the likely lads. 'Oh *!@#,' he said. 'We've just been passed by *!@#-ing Kerre Woodham!' A bad day had just got a whole lot worse — a gorgeous fit young thing had been left in the dust by an overweight boiler from the 'burbs. Yes! Score one for the old ladies! When you're running a marathon to finish, not to race, it really doesn't matter what time you do. But you'll find that you set yourself little targets along the way and play little games — like, if I don't look at my watch until the next telephone box I pass, I can have another dinosaur lolly. Like, I'll take those two boys up ahead and they can suffer the horror of watching Pure Indulgence disappear into the distance in front of them.

The last bridge loomed up ahead before we hit the CBD. It's only a small hump of a bridge, but at the tail end of a marathon, it loomed like Everest. Di and John were waiting right at that critical point and their encouragement gave me the strength to crawl up the hill. Then it was the red railings of the Port, which have always seemed to stretch on forever and the sight of the clock tower on the Harbour Buildings. Bruce checked his watch and told me we were doing fine. We could come in under 4:30, he said. Whatever, I puffed, but like a weary horse, I could scent that we were almost home. One km to go, and we were nearly there. We wound our way through the streets of the Viaduct. So very close now and it would all be over. And there it was. Victoria Park, with the tunnel to the finish line at the end lined with a cheering crowd. The clock above the finish line showed 4:29.

'Dig deep,' yelled Bruce. 'We've got to get under 4:30.'

'I have dug deep,' I wailed back.

'I need more,' he said.

'There *is* no more,' I puffed out.

'Put your bloody head down and *run!*' Bruce yelled. And I did. After 4 hours and 29 minutes of running, I put down my head and I ran. The seconds ticked by, the cheering faces passed in a blur and then we were there. Over the finish line, in just under 4 hours and 30 minutes and Gaz was there and the Irishman was there and Kate was there, with her boyfriend. I hugged them all and thanked them all and I couldn't stop grinning. I was absolutely euphoric. There is nothing quite like it, other than perhaps childbirth. Without a doubt, it's a monumental physical effort, but it's not just the run on the day. It's getting up early on a weekend morning for the long run when all you want to do is curl up under the covers. It's getting out there when it's cold and dark and persisting down with rain. It's the hours spent pounding the pavements, and the times you've forced yourself to keep going when all you want to do is run into the nearest café and get the staff to pour you a stonking great chardonnay.

There were interviews to do afterwards, and the photo that was published in the *New Zealand Herald* the morning after the event summed up exactly how I felt. In this case, a picture did indeed tell a thousand words and I ordered a copy of it, which I have framed to remind me that I have the tenacity and strength of mind to run a marathon, so therefore there is no reason at all why I can't accept and conquer other challenges that come my way. After the interviews, I had to present myself at the adidas Sports medicine tent as we marathon runners were part of an experiment in water loss. We'd been weighed when we collected our race packs, and we were weighed again after the race, before we'd headed off to be fed and watered. I couldn't believe when I stood on the scales that I hadn't lost a gram. 'These must be faulty,' I said to the young doctor supervising the information gathering. 'No, they're not,' he assured me, 'and besides, it's good that you've maintained the same weight. It means you kept your fluids up all the way round.' Reassuring news for a finely honed athlete. Not such good news for an overweight woman in her forties who was hoping to have a couple of days of ravaged thinness as a reward for running such a long way.

Antonia from Pead PR and Alex from the Cystic Fibrosis Association were waiting in a marquee for me and it was a good feeling to hand over a cheque for $5000 to Alex. It was a very rewarding exercise on a personal level, but to have been the catalyst for the donation to be made felt good as well. We chatted for a while and then I went over to Les Mills to shower and change and scarf down some lunch before Gaz and I went to see Murray Deaker at NewsTalkZB for a post-marathon interview.

Murray had done the Auckland Marathon some years previously and he'd hated every bloody moment of it. It took him more than six hours — in fact, he took so long that the race marshals were driving in front of him picking up the orange cones from the road as he slugged it out towards the end. He thought I was absolutely mad and Muzz being Muzz, he didn't hold back in telling me the horror stories. Bless him, though, he took an interest and he gave us an hour on his nationwide afternoon talk show following the marathon. I wanted Gaz to get the kudos and credit he deserved for getting me across that finish line. And not only getting me across, but getting me across in one piece and with a net time of 4:26:33. The fact that I'd enjoyed it was a bonus. I promise you, there was not one moment where I was in pain or desperation. Those people who do a marathon tough, like Murray and like Mary, who ran the Rotorua Marathon in pouring rain with a crippling period that started 10 km in, have my utmost admiration. I don't know how long I could have endured if I'd been fighting a sore foot or a pain in my side. It's a long way to go not having a good time. Those who take the longest but finish anyway are truly heroic. Anyway, Gaz and I sat with Murray for an hour, taking calls, and at the end of the hour, Murray said to me that he was very impressed and that he thought differently of me now.

'What? I'm not the flighty tart you thought I was?' I said.

'Exactly!' he said with a laugh. You'll find that people respond one of two ways when you tell them you've run a marathon. It's either appalled incomprehension (those who haven't run one) or complete and utter admiration (those who have). You have become a member of a small and very exclusive club and you have every right to be damn proud of yourself.

After the interview with Murray, the Irishman and I headed over to Devonport to pick up my gear. Then it was home for a blob out on the couch before heading out to Prego to pick up a takeout pizza. Once we got home, we opened the bottle of Wither Hills pinot I'd bought all those months ago in Blenheim, where I'd barely made it round the half. I toasted my Irishman and thanked him for all his support and he toasted me. I felt utterly content. I'd done something I would never have thought possible. All those hours out on the street; all those early morning wake-up calls; all the stress; all the worry — it was worth it. I'd discovered a lot about what my body could and couldn't do, and what I needed to do to keep it healthy. More importantly, I'd discovered how strong my willpower was when I needed it to be. Some of my friends pointed out that I'd given up drinking for seven years and surely that took more willpower, but it was different. I didn't *want* to drink, so not drinking was easy. Omission is so much easier than commission. As in giving up is easier than doing. I really, really didn't want to run on so many occasions and yet I'd forced myself out the door, and nine times out of ten, I enjoyed it once I was out there. I'd made some amazing new friends and found out just how supportive good friends could be. It had been one hell of an experience and now it was over. I would plan another challenge, but for now, I would just bask in the joy of knowing I would never again have to get up at 6 a.m. on a rainy Saturday and run for hours. I polished off the last of the pizza, gave a satisfied belch, and poured another pinot. Life didn't get much better than this.

GAZ

I remember receiving a call from Antonia from Pead PR, the company that seemed to act more like Kerre's Angels than a PR company.

'Gaz,' said Antonia, 'could you do me a favour and accompany Kerre to pick up her race pack. She seems to be a little worked up about the race.'

I joined Kerre the day after her little incident with the Panic Fairy to pick up her race pack and realised just how mentally draining the unknown can be. Throughout my life I've competed in various races and I'm used to the hype and excitement involved and take it for granted and just deal with it. But seeing Kerre that day made me realise how big a deal it is for a first-time runner to compete. You don't have to be told about fear, you can pick it up from the environment around you. That's exactly what happened to Kerre — the registration scene hit home hard as the enormity of the event dawned on her.

There is no getting around the fact that your first major event will be the scariest, but in my eyes it's all a part of it and makes the accomplishment that much sweeter.

Of course, if you are well prepared, you will find it a lot easier to cope with the situation and you won't have a pre-race meltdown. Here are a few simple tips on race prep and race day:

- Always go along to registration with a friend or fellow runner to pick up your race pack.
- Drive the course the day before or, if you can, run a section of it a week before.

- Write a list of the gear you will need for the race, bullet point the items and check them off the morning before the big race.
- Don't worry if you don't get enough sleep the night before. The adrenalin flows through the body from the time you get up and doesn't stop until you cross the finish line. This is enought to forget about the lack of sleep. Just don't plan on going out that night!

The marathon day itself should be an experience of a lifetime. You've done all the training and, if you've done it properly, the largest week of your training will actually feel harder than the race itself. By the time the race has come around you will have had approximately 36 weeks of training, brought your running up to 80 km a week and put in a longest run of at least 32 km. Two weeks before the race you will taper and, as a result, by race day you'll feel fresh and bursting out of your running shoes ready to go. Add in the hype of the day and you've got all the ingredients for a great experience. I've always said, if I can get my client to the start line with enough kilometres under their belt and in a well-rested state, then they will definitely finish the race.

With a race as long as the marathon, it's a great idea to break it down into smaller chunks, even if you only want to finish it. This is called working out your splits. It helps you not to go out too quickly and keeps you on an even pace over the race. Once you've got your first marathon under your belt, you may find you want to do others, and working out your splits will help you improve your time. And I have yet to come across a runner who doesn't want to beat their personal best.

Splits are like pizza slices — you wouldn't eat a whole pizza in one mouthful, and likewise, don't tackle the marathon in one piece. Divide it up into eight 5 km sections and one little bit of 2.2 km. This helps the distance become realistic and attainable. Work out your goal time, e.g. 4:30:00, and then calculate what time will have elapsed by each of your split markers if you run at the pace needed to achieve your goal time. I get my clients to work out two sets of splits — one their actual goal time and the other the time they might go for if they were feeling great on the day. Here's an example:

Split	Goal time 4:30:00 Time	Great time 4:15:00 Time
5 km	0:31	0:30
10 km	1:02	1:00
15 km	1:33	1:30
20 km	2:04	2:00
25 km	2:35	2:30
30 km	3:06	3:00
35 km	3:37	3:30
40 km	4:08	4:00
42.2 km	4:30	4:15

Note that I have allowed a little buffer time between the 40 km and the end. This allows you to savour the moment, wave and high-five everyone down the finish chute!

The two target times are 15 minutes apart as at this level of marathon running quarter-hour markers are the target barriers and milestones that people try to beat. If you are right-handed, then have your 'goal time' splits in your right hand, and keep your 'great time' splits in your left hand. Reverse it if you are left-handed. It's more natural to look at your dominant hand, so you should hold your realistic splits in this hand and only consult the other splits if everything is going exceptionally well at the halfway point, otherwise you may find yourself hitting a wall at the 32 km mark.

After I had been working with Kerre for a while I had a feeling she could go under 4:30:00, but I was honestly expecting her to finish in closer to five hours. Through her dedication to training and stubbornness in the race, and her consistency of pace, she pulled out a great result. It was even more amazing since her longest training run was a bit on the short side. Not everyone can get away with this, but Kerre seems to work better under pressure. I always referred to her as a diesel tractor . . . she'll run all day on a sniff of diesel, but you can't let her run out of fuel or break down, because you may never get her going again!

chapter seven

Releasing my inner packhorse

That would have been a good place to end my story. A 'How to Run a Marathon' guide should start with the desire of a person to do so, move through the training, and culminate in a stupendously climactic breasting of the finish-line tape. But oh no. Not this one. Buoyed by the euphoria that I hadn't died, Gaz persuaded me that running the New York Marathon would be a good idea. Everyone does one marathon he said. You've got to do two. And New York is one of the great marathons to run. OK, I said. Let's. It's the same sort of ridiculous endorphin rush you get after childbirth. You immediately forget the discomfort and the inconvenience and the pain, and holding that baby in your arms, you proclaim that you'll have ten of the little critters.

When Gaz suggested the New York Marathon, I was filled with desire. My training partners, Mary and Lee and Lavina, had come back raving about what an experience it was. My colleague at NewsTalkZB, Larry Williams, who's run quite a few marathons, including New York, concurred.

He told me New Yorkers lined the streets, five deep, for the whole 42 km and if there was any chance at all of running it, I should take it. And so, stupidly, foolishly, I signed up to run New York.

Gaz had decided to take a team across — there would be ten of us and so we reserved ten places on a package tour to the marathon and set about finding nine other suckers who would run it too.

I asked my lovely friend Jo to come with me. She had been enormously supportive of my decision to run Auckland and I thought it would be a marvellous challenge for her. She's an incredibly capable, competent woman, a television producer, wife and young mother, and if anyone could fit in the training, she could. Except that her body wasn't cut out to run marathons. That's the good thing about deciding to undertake a massive physical challenge. You find out all sorts of things about yourself. And when Jo went through the prelim checks, she found that she was hypermobile and that running would totally dislocate her limbs. So she was out. And that was a huge disappointment for her. Once you decide in your mind you're going to run a marathon, you're already halfway there. To be told it's just not physically possible is enormously disappointing. And that might happen to you. It's OK. Endure the disappointment and take up another challenge.

For Jo, it was starting a new business. She's not the sort of girl to sit around wondering what might have been. And that's the right attitude to take. If marathon running is not for you, take up swimming. Or enrol in a Maori language programme. Or take a wine appreciation course. Whatever. If you feel like you need a challenge, find one that suits your physical capabilities and your lifestyle.

I really didn't feel the need to run another marathon. I hope I've stressed to you how much effort and time is required to run the bloody things. There is no way to short circuit the training. But the team Gaz had assembled would be running to raise money for the Breast Cancer Research Trust and that's a very worthy cause and I'd paid the non-refundable deposit to the travel agent and, besides, I'd agreed to write a book about marathon running and between Gaz and the publishers, it was decided that running the New York Marathon would be a great part of the story. So it was back into training. But this time my body decided it had had enough.

I was rehearsing the Farmers fashion parade one hot Friday in February. It was an all-day affair and I was MCing two shows — one for the fashion media and one later in the evening for Farmers' customers. There was a lot of standing around and the cramping pain in my back was getting more and more difficult to ignore. To the consternation of the Farmers chaps, I told them to carry on chatting to me but if they didn't mind, I'd just lie on the ground while they talked. Who lies about on the ground? Drunks do. Homeless people do. Highly paid professional MCs shouldn't. But there was nothing I could do about it. I was even beginning to doubt my ability to do the shows. I'd never, ever had back pain before, but it was bloody agony.

I walked with crab steps, hunched over, out to the back where the models were getting changed and retrieved my phone from my bag. I dialled Gaz — I'd had quite a session with him the day before working on my glutes to strengthen me up for running and I wondered if I'd triggered something with the exercise. Mercifully, he was free and he biked straight down to see me. Ten minutes later, I was lying flat on my stomach with Gaz straddling me, one elbow grinding into the small of my back while he received instructions from a physio friend of his. All around us, half-naked visions of loveliness were undressing and shimmying into teeny-tiny scraps of lace for the lingerie section of the show.

'Of all the girls in the room you could be straddling, you end up with the overweight forty-two-year-old,' I sniggered to Gaz.

'Don't,' he sighed. 'It will just make me bitter.'

Thanks to Gaz's not-so-tender ministrations, I was able to get up and walk, and although my back was uncomfortable, at least it had stopped the paralysing cramps. I did the two shows, and a good time was had by all. But clearly, there was something very wrong with my body. Although I'd pulled up just fine after the marathon, the running had taken its toll. I was in the very position I'd tried so hard not to end up in — just another clapped-out runner. It was frustrating and infuriating.

I could barely walk over the next few weeks, and there was no thought of me running. The New York group would meet up for runs around Auckland's waterfront, and off the fit young things would go — pert buttocks bouncing off into the distance. It was ages before I saw any of their faces: all I knew of my team-mates was the backs of their heads and the shapes of their bums, as I walked — slowly — behind them.

Gaz decided that along with the walking I would benefit from Pilates and instructed me to get along and see a mate of his called Ree. I had always dismissed Pilates as the preserve of the yummy mummy set — those women whose job it is to look good and manage a beautiful home. If I was going to exercise, I wanted to get hot and sweaty and get my heart rate up — not sit there squeezing and contracting in an ever-so genteel and ladylike fashion. But Ree was also a physio, so I said I'd give it a go. And I have to tell you — if you decide to run a marathon, get yourself along for Pilates sessions. I'm a total convert. It helps when you have an instructor as wonderful as Ree to get you started, but from what I've seen, there appear to be very few dud instructors. They're all lovely and seem to be very well trained in this country.

Pilates for runners makes perfect sense. If you're going to run, you have to work on your core strength. I'd been running with a wiggly bum — my hips swung backwards and forwards putting an intolerable strain on my lower back. I've always had a wiggly bottom — my daughter's dad used to say I walked like I should have a whole line of ducklings trailing after me. Gaz had tried to build up my stomach muscles, but they were so weak and pathetic, my back hurt after just a few exercises, and besides, the focus really was on running. I'd run 42 km with a weak stomach and now I was pretty much buggered. It was going to take lots of time, lots of recuperation and lots of massage to build me back up again.

There was a further complicating factor in that I was booked to take a three-week cruise round the Mediterranean in August. It was work, in that I was leading a tour group, but really, there's work, and there's work, isn't there? While I was studying journalism at Wellington Polytechnic a million years ago, I'd earned money at various jobs, including working at the local fish and chip shop, and cleaning flash people's houses. Reeking of animal fat and scrubbing crud that is not your own off toilet bowls is not in the same category of work as taking a group of lovely, intelligent, broad-minded people on a tour around Italy aboard a five-masted sailing ship. Especially when I didn't actually have to do the hard work of knowing where to go or what to do. There was a highly trained and competent professional to do that. No, I just had to bound around like an excitable Labrador, ensuring everyone was happy and entertained. And while that all sounded perfectly pleasant, it would not be conducive to good training for a marathon.

The ship we were to sail on was small and perfectly formed. It wasn't one of those great big monsters that cross the ocean. She was tiny and I couldn't possibly run around her as part of my training. I'd have been like a gerbil on a wheel. She did have a gym, so I would have to use that — when I wasn't eating, drinking and bounding.

Gaz despaired. Here we were in February, the New York Marathon was in November, I couldn't actually run and I was facing a long recuperation period and even if I did get back up running, I would have three weeks off right when I should be peaking in my training. On the plus side, I'd run a marathon before, so I had a base fitness — I wasn't starting totally from scratch — and Gaz said I had superior mental fitness which would enable me to overcome my physical deficiencies in a way no ordinary mortal could. Not in so many words. He actually said I was as tough as old boots and as stubborn as an old packhorse, but I'm sure I interpreted his words correctly.

Eventually I could run again. And that's the thing with injuries. If you get to them early enough, and you allow enough time, you will run again. If you want to. Of course, you could always take the injury as a sign, retire early and give up on the whole stupid idea, but come on, people. Toughen up. You surely don't think your underworked, overweight, middle-aged carcass is going to be expected to start heavy physical exercise without clapping out in some way, do you? Every runner gets an injury somewhere along the line. The secret is to recognise the signs early and allow the injury time to heal. You have to be tough but not too tough, because if you run through an injury, you can actually do some serious damage.

So there I was back running and the Taupo Half-marathon was looming. In comparison to my attitude before the Woodbourne Half, I was completely sanguine.

A large part of marathon running is getting over the fear of the unknown. A couple of our group hadn't actually run a half before and they were putting themselves under all sorts of pressure. They didn't know that they could run 21 km — they'd never done it before, and so their subconscious was playing all sorts of tricks on them. They'd done the training; Gaz assured them that they were ready, but until they'd actually run the distance they couldn't be certain they would get through. The plan was that we would all drive down to Taupo, share a meal together and stay at one hotel. It would a good chance for the ten members of the New York Marathon team to bond, and for me, it would be a good chance to see some of my team members' faces for the first time, given that I'd been eating their dust for the past three months.

Kamilla, one of the New York team members, was driving her Get Shorty wagon down to Taupo, so three of us decided to travel with her. The people-mover was nicknamed the Mothership as Kamilla's a busy working mum of two and it was well specced out for our journey. We had endless bags of lollies, the latest girly magazines and after a quick stop-off in Tirau, a little bottle of Lindauer each — just to help with the carb loading. Actually, this is probably a good place to introduce you to the Mission:Possible team. I've been wondering how to fit them into the narrative, but given that I'll be referring to these people constantly from here on in, you need to know who they are. I guess now's as good a time as any for you to meet my fellow New York marathoners.

Jean-Michel Tallot is a gorgeous young man, impeccably mannered, a very, very good runner and Gaz's partner in crime. A natural athlete, he'd always wanted to run a marathon and given that cancer had affected his family, he was keen to run for the cause.

Steven Fair had run three marathons already, was built like a whippet and was a good running mate for JM.

Olivia Jeffrey — Livvy — is the perfect woman. Just under 2 metres tall — three-quarters of that leg — organised, a whiz at fundraising and PR — she and Gaz were formidable when it came to finding sponsors and making things happen. She could also run like the wind, but then, when you're built like a racehorse, you should be able to.

Angela Daniel is a gorgeous wee blonde whose partner Lachie was a big part of the team as well. Although Ange looks like a beautiful accessory herself, she actually makes a very healthy living *creating* beautiful accessories. She's a jeweller and her empire is growing by the year. As well as training for the marathon, she was fitting in her two existing shops and managed to open a third. A wee dynamo.

Geeling Ching is a fabulous foodie — she's the manager of Soul Bistro and Bar at the Viaduct and has been in the restaurant business for years, in between modelling and acting. Those of us who are refugees from the eighties will remember her best as David Bowie's little China girl in the video of the same song. She's a natural runner and as her mother was a breast cancer survivor, she was keen to help fundraise for the BCRT.

Nick Bryant is a fabulous father of two with a sizzler of a wife. He feared that, although he'd played sports all his life, his body was starting to pack up and unless he got his A into G, he would suffer a physical decline. The marathon was his attempt to get his health back on track.

Kamilla Andersson is a single mum of two small children, the owner of her own business, and a single-minded, generous, determined soul. She ran the Auckland Marathon pretty much on her own, the same year I did it, and how she manages to fit all she does into a day, as well as the training, is beyond me. I could never achieve in a week what she does in a day. She's an inspiration.

Blair Huston is a forty-year-old successful businessman who was very close to his dad. The two boys had always wanted to do three things together: walk the Milford Track, get their private pilot's licence and run a marathon. Unfortunately, Blair's dad died before they could accomplish their goals and now Blair was ticking off the boxes for him. Blair was our man of mystery. As one of Auckland's most eligible bachelors, he very seldom made the Saturday morning runs — in fact, he turned up for fewer than I did! — but he had a secret training programme that he was sticking to. You don't get to be as successful as Blair without having willpower and determination.

Hilary Lewis is a delight. She had had an operation on her legs when she was little and, according to Gaz, she shouldn't have been walking, far less running a marathon. She travelled a lot with her job as e-commerce director for the House of Travel and had to do her runs on her own in Russia, London and the south of France, to name just a few places. She was a joy to travel with and one of the gutsiest runners in our group.

And then there's me — but you know quite enough about me and my motivation for running the marathon already.

It was hosing down in Taupo when we arrived and the run across from the car park to the registration hall almost knackered a couple of us. We were puffed and gasping for breath after the 250-metre run and the newbies — those who'd never run a marathon before — were terrified. If we can't run this far, how the hell are we going to manage 21 km? they wailed. Again, this is completely normal. Remember me just before Woodbourne? Gaz got me to warm up by running the length of a football field and back and I thought I was going to get the stitch. It's a combination of nerves and your body preparing itself for the real battle that lies ahead. It knows it's got a huge struggle in front of it — all your resources will kick in then. In the meantime, you're on your own.

After registration, we checked into our hotel and prepared for dinner. Gaz had organised a high-carb meal with the hotel and it was great sitting round with thirty or so people, all with the same goal in mind. However, at about 9 p.m. people started drifting away. Ah well, they said, must head off. Big day tomorrow. And within half an hour, two-thirds of the room was gone. All in bed by 9.30! And these were grown-ups! Not members of the Sacred Heart Girls College marathon team. Although judging by the glint in a couple of my fellow runners' single and wandering eyes, they weren't going to bed to rest.

Given that I normally hit the hay around 1 a.m., and have done so every night for the past twenty years, there was no way I was heading up to my room. I'd have ended up lying there, staring at the ceiling for hours. I was able to inveigle a couple of runners — and Gaz — to stay with me while I chucked another couple of red wines down my throat, but eventually I was forced to concede defeat and retire to bed. A couple of my fellow runners were a little concerned at my propping up the bar the night before the run, but my body was used to alcohol and I was drinking plenty of water as well. Anyway, it was only a half. I slept like a lamb and woke to a perfect day for running.

The rain had cleared and the day dawned clear and bright. We boarded the Mothership and Kamilla steered us down to the car park where we were to start the half. We had four hundred sausages with us, ten bags of onions and about twenty loaves of bread, courtesy of the Mad Butcher, bless him. A big part of the New York Marathon team effort was raising money for the Breast Cancer Research Trust and our first fundraising initiative was a sausage sizzle after the half. Mercifully, the running team wasn't going to have to stand for hours on our tortured tootsies burning bangers — we had a team of volunteers who'd donated their time to sell the sossies on our behalf.

We staggered over with our booty and found our tent that the boys had erected in an impressively quick time. The tent had been donated, too. It's amazing how generous people can be when they know you're trying to raise money for a good cause.

There are endless worthy causes and you can't walk down the street or dash into your local supermarket without being accosted by some fresh-faced, doe-eyed beauty, all firm youth and velvety skin who wants to talk to you earnestly about the plight of the whales and how just $10 can take an impoverished child in an African village and transform them into a Nobel Prize-winning writer. They always look at you askance when you say you have no cash on you. I know they don't believe me. They think I'm just a bloated member of the bourgeoisie who's too mean to part with a shilling and mark me down as the first to go against the wall come the revolution. But it's true. As any parent of a teenager can attest, you never have cash once you have kids. Paul Holmes has a T-shirt with a slogan that reads 'The Incredible Dad — see money disappear'.

However, I digress. People's generosity is a truly remarkable thing. And we were blessed that our team — Mission:Possible — had been able to call upon the kindness of so many strangers. We dumped the sausages, admired the tent, and headed for the start line. The start was staggered and Kamilla and I stuck together so we could at least begin the run together. It is a rare and wonderful thing to find someone who can run at your pace. I admired the Titirangi Tunnel Rats, who seemed to be able to run at any pace with anyone. I simply can't do that. I go at one speed — 10 km an hour, give or take the odd minute, and that's it.

From the time I took my first step in Taupo, I was in trouble. Every now and then, on my long runs and this was right back when I first started running, I'd get a pain in my foot. Right under the second toe, on the ball of my foot, an ache would start up after an hour, which would intensify so that it felt like a burning poker being forced into my foot — without wishing to overdramatise the situation. It fricking hurt and I could set my watch by it. I'd feel the pain, check my watch and whaddaya know? An hour's gone by. But this time, on this morning, the pain began with the first step. And that had never happened before. I tried to distract myself by using the power of positive thinking — my foot is *not* hurting; imagine how much more pain some people are in; aren't you lucky being able to be here today — but you know, when your foot hurts and you have to run on it and you've only done 3 km and there are 18 to go, it's not much fun.

As we left the main road heading out of Taupo and ran towards the lake, I asked Kamilla how she was feeling.

'Good,' she replied.

'Does anything hurt?' I asked.

'*Everything* hurts!' she snapped. 'Thanks for reminding me!'

It is very poor form to mention sore body parts while out running. It is generally accepted that everyone is in some sort of pain and discomfort and there is no reason why your particular pain deserves special mention. It saps confidence and lowers morale. So I shut up, put my head down and tried to go to my happy place.

It's a nice Half, Taupo. For a while. You start at the big park in the middle of town, head out round the lake, up the hill, across a farm, and back round the lake to home. Easy. Except it's not. Taupo can be deceptively difficult. The weather is changeable year on year. We were fortunate that the rain cleared and it was a fine, sunny day without being too hot. People who've run Taupo in other years have told me that they almost had to pull out with exposure; others said they were in grave danger of getting sunstroke. Although I sound like an A-grade moaner, what I'm saying is that it's very hard to predict exactly what sort of weather you're going to get, so that's why it pays to run in all conditions. When you're sitting at home having a pitched battle with yourself about whether you should go running — It's dreadful outside! What's the point of going running only to get pneumonia? No, I'll give it a miss today and make up for it tomorrow — remind yourself that this is all good practice for the real thing.

But back to the Taupo Half. There was a mental setback when I realised that, although I'd reached the farm that was the start of the journey back into town, we had to run a meaningless couple of ks down a suburban street before going through the farm gate to make up the distance. This is where the mental toughness is so important, as it can really knock you around if you feel swindled and cheated. As it was, I focused on all the good folk of Taupo who'd taken the time to come out and cheer on neighbours, friends and complete strangers, and the wee kids in their pyjamas who were offering water were so cute it would have been a fearful crime to have snarled at them in my frustration, so all was well. The field itself was uneven terrain and a lot of the runners were a bit grumpy about that. They were used to running on asphalt. I'd had the benefit of a few runs with the Tunnel Rats in the Waitakere hills, so the dirt path didn't faze me so much. But again, if you're not used to something, it makes it that much tougher to stick it out running when you're starting to tire.

We came out of the paddock and headed back round the lake towards town. My foot was really hurting now and although the random chap running alongside me who told me to 'Just tell yourself that it's not sore' was only trying to help, I had to refrain from belting him. I knew better. The bloody thing *was* sore, had been sore since the gun, and would no doubt continue to be sore until the finish. I hadn't seen Gaz at this stage, so began muttering to myself about how he was undoubtedly favouring the fast runners, and was probably enjoying a drink with the cool young ones who'd already finished — mumble, grumble, bitch and moan — when I came round a corner and there he was, parked on his bike at the 16 km mark, loaded up with Gatorade and jelly dinosaurs. He asked me how I was doing, I told him my foot hurt and he told me it wasn't far till the end. Seeing him perked me up no end, far more so than the Gatorade or the sugar hit in the lollies. Knowing that somebody cares enough to hang around and cheer you is enormously important to marathon runners. We're needy little critters.

I spent the next couple of ks blessing Gaz in my mind and reminding myself how mind-numbingly dull it must be for him to stand by the side of a lake for a couple of hours and watch runners go by. There was a head wind coming into town, which made the last part of the run a little more difficult, but finally I could see the park ahead and knew that there was only a few more metres to go. Round the corner, just a few more minutes — and there was the biggest, steepest hill I had ever seen in my life. The last few steps of a tough half-marathon and you're expected to scale a bloody mountain? I was furious, as indeed were the other runners, new to Taupo, who were around me. We wasted valuable breath muttering and cursing as we scaled the thing and there it was. The finish chute to the end.

I crossed the line and immediately took off my shoes to release my throbbing foot. There was nothing to see, and I knew as soon as I stopped running it would come right. I made my way back to our tent, which was miraculously still standing, and waited my turn for a massage. Karen, who ran the massage clinic, and Ree, our physio/Pilates instructor, had kindly volunteered to come down for the day and give us post-run massages, and although experts seem to be divided as to whether there are any real recovery benefits in having massages immediately after races, I can assure you that runners are unequivocal in their belief that a post-run massage is just the thing. We watched jealously as those already on the tables sighed and groaned under the tender ministrations of the two skilled practitioners and kept a watchful eye on the time to ensure nobody got more than their fair share and we weren't cheated out of a single second of bliss.

We were truly blessed with the weather as the heavens opened just as the prize-giving began. We decided to load up the vehicles and head back to Auckland, well pleased with our away trip. The journey home was a heck of a lot quieter than the trip down on Friday, that's for sure. I was pleased I'd been able to run the Taupo Half, because at the beginning of the year, I didn't think I'd be able to run again. I'd only had a short lead-in time, but I guess there was some residual fitness from my training for the Auckland Marathon. I did exactly the same time as I did for Woodbourne — 2:03 — but I felt no real sense of achievement and I still didn't feel particularly inspired about New York. Especially if I was going to have to run for four and a half hours with a throbbing foot. Although I loved hanging out with my other runners and was enjoying the social aspect of the training, I really didn't have my heart in it. And that makes marathon training so much tougher.

GAZ

The recovery phase after the marathon is very important. Your immediate priority is to drink sufficient liquid to correct any dehydration and salt losses that may have occurred. You may crave salt after a race, and if so it is fine to eat salty foods such as potato chips. A runner's appetite may be suppressed for a few hours after a marathon, and when it returns (and don't worry, it will!) there is usually a craving for high-fat or high-protein foods. Enjoy this time and celebrate your running victory!

The day after the race is usually characterised by varying degrees of mental and physical fatigue. Your legs will feel stiff, often for 48 hours after the run. You'll find the simplest set of stairs seems like Mount Everest and getting out of a car seems to take an eternity. You'll almost feel like trading the vehicle in for a Zimmer frame! Not to fear, this is normal and it's just the body's way of getting rid of the build-up of toxins and repairing damaged muscle fibres. It's always a good idea to get a 10-minute 'flush-out' massage straight after your race, then follow that with a full-hour massage a couple of days later.

The week after the marathon usually requires some down time and a complete rest from running. Often the mere thought of running conjures bad memories and you may experience a sense of anticlimax now that you have achieved your goal. My advice is just to ride it out — within a couple of weeks you'll only remember the great times during the race and find yourself thinking about the next challenge.

There are many conflicting theories on when you should run your next marathon. From personal experience, I like to see my less-experienced runners tackle only one marathon per year. As they get stronger, they can increase this number. It's important to stress that the body needs rest as much as it does training, and by allowing enough time it will adapt to the rigours of distance running so that you can compete more frequently.

I was excited to hear that Kerre was keen to go to New York, even though she took a little bit of persuading. I was beside myself. It's not often you get to be a part of the largest marathon in the world. The team was picked, we joined partnerships with the Breast Cancer Research Trust and I enlisted the help of a close friend and savvy businesswoman, Olivia Jeffrey. She wanted to run the New York Marathon and had a few friends who were interested. Before we knew it the team was full. This new breed of runners had disposable incomes and enjoyed a glass of champagne. I was excited by this prospect and looked forward to the coming months.

With everything in place, Kerre and I were off on another journey. But this time it was a little different for her. I could see it in her training as we came up to the Taupo Half — she just didn't seem to be as involved as the first time around. I think it comes down to what's on the line. Kerre had promised to a small child that she would run the Auckland Marathon for her and you never renege on that! Even though we were to support another great charity, it just wasn't as personal to her and that brings up a great point. Make sure you make the marathon personal. Take on a charity that you relate to and make yourself personally accountable. It works!

chapter eight

More indulgence

To complicate matters, as I've mentioned, the Irishman and I were set to take a cruise in the Mediterranean in August. Every year since I'd started on NewsTalkZB I'd been asked to escort a tour. Initially, the idea appealed. What's not to like? I love people, I love travelling, I love the idea of doing so at next to no cost. However, after I'd agreed early on when I'd first started at ZB to take a trip to India, and the travel agent disappeared with all the loot from an earlier tour, I was reluctant to take one on. Mercifully, all my people got their deposits back, but what if they hadn't? Although I wouldn't be legally responsible, I would have felt morally responsible and I didn't want to spend the rest of my life in servitude paying back people for a crime I hadn't committed. 'But he was so charming!' I wailed to the salesman who gave me the bad news that Willie had done a runner. 'Well, yeah,' said the salesman, who'd taken a bath. 'Con men usually are. It's a prerequisite for the job.'

So understandably, I was wary of signing up for another

tour that carried my name. However, ten years later and a gorgeous bubbly blonde rang me at home. I didn't, of course, know she was blonde at the time. That knowledge came later. What she did offer was a trip around the Med, backed by an international tour group. No thank you, I said snippily. I've been offered tours before and I'll tell you what I tell them all — no thank you. She laughed and said this one was something special. They all say that, I responded. Well, can I send you the promotional material, she replied, nothing daunted. If you must, I snapped, just this side of civil. I had absolutely no intention of taking three weeks' leave to escort a bunch of grumpy old farts around the Mediterranean. And besides, what would we do with the dog?

However, seconds after I received the brochure in the mail, I was on the phone to the gorgeous Jacqueline. I had imagined some huge floating factory that caters for thousands. This was a five-masted sailing ship that took 180. The *Wind Surf* was absolutely beautiful. She sailed from Rome to Venice via Corfu and Croatia and there was a week in Venice to recover from the rigours of five-star luxury. What's a girl to do? She's to get on the phone to the travel agent, that's what she's to do. You know when I said no, Jacqueline? I said. I really meant yes. That's what they all say, she said with a laugh and signed me up to a three-week Mediterranean cruise in the middle of August 2007.

Which is all very well and good and fabulous, when you're being signed up in August 2006, but all of a sudden the embarkation date was looming, and I had a marathon to run. Even if I'd had the best of intentions, there was no way a three-week tour of the Med was going to involve intensive marathon training. And I didn't have the best of intentions at all. In fact, I thought if I managed to get my fat arse off the deck chair for ten minutes a day I'd be doing well. And the food! How was I going to negotiate the nutritional minefield? No thank you, I won't have the cocktail/red wine/pâté/pasta because I'm running a marathon in two months? I don't think so. I could have been run down by a car while crossing the road. Or slipped on the deck while bringing in the washing. Or discovered I had a brain tumour. All of which have resulted in the deaths of people I know who had no idea they were about to cark it. So you might as well have a good time, because most of us aren't here for a long one. Which may well be a fine philosophy if you're not running a marathon, but I was. Gaz gave me a training programme that he pretended I would follow, and I accepted the training programme and lied through my teeth and said I would follow it to the letter and we both went away, shaking our heads and thinking it would be a miracle if I made it to the start line of the New York Marathon, far less the finish.

I'd been to see yet another expert, who told me my left leg was a good few millimetres longer than my right and that was what was causing the pain and gave me a set of breathing exercises to do to fix it. I didn't bother. If you decide to run a marathon and you have the time, the money and the energy to visit experts, you'll get lots of advice from lovely, well-meaning people who believe in their philosophy and want to help you get to the finish. Don't take it all. Take what makes sense to you, and works for you. For me, lying on the floor, moving my elbows and knees to make up for the lack of formative crawling I'd done as a baby, didn't work for me. What did work was a young podiatrist, recommended to me by the Pilates team, who agreed that my leg was gimpy but gave me an insole to put in the shoe to correct the imbalance. And what's more, he told me that he didn't want to be paid unless it worked. Can you believe it? I loved him. So I took the insole away with me, and said I'd try it when I went for runs in Italy. I knew I wouldn't be running far, if I ran at all, so I couldn't do much damage. There's a real danger when you try insoles that you're trying to instantly correct something that's taken thirty or forty years to build up, so podiatrists always tell you to start slowly. Don't go galloping off on three-hour runs with new insoles. No danger there — I was about to head off on holiday.

And marvellous it was, too. The Irishman, who takes some persuading to leave his castle in Grey Lynn, and the dog both conceded we had struck house-sitter Lotto with the bloke who was moving in while we were away. He was a Welsh policeman on a working holiday — was a friend of a friend — who was sleeping on a couch, so grateful for a real bed and he loved dogs. Score! I didn't have to worry about the house, the dog or a fretting Irishman. I only had to worry about doing the best job I could for our travellers.

But again, I'd struck gold. The people on the tour were absolutely gorgeous — sophisticated, open-minded, independent darlings, many of whom had travelled before. We all clicked so well we were asked on numerous occasions if we were a family reunion. It was just great — the weather was perfect, the ship was heaven, the food was exquisite and the wine was plentiful. And I managed three — count them: three — runs in three weeks.

The first was just after we arrived in Rome. Jetlagged to buggery I decided to use the hours that I was spending looking at the 16th-century ceiling of my bedroom, which had no doubt been looked at before, to go for a run. It was the last Sunday in August — the weekend before Romans head back to town after their summer holidays — so the city was unbelievably quiet. I headed off, with no clear route in mind other than a vague desire to head towards the Colosseum. Down the main drag I jogged, up to the great white wedding cake that is the Monument to Victor Emmanuel, up the stairs and then down past the ruins of the Forum. I stopped to take a drink of water that flowed from a tap in the wall and wondered if thousands of years ago, Roman senators had done the same. Probably not. It was likely that the plumbing had been put in by some pot-bellied, comb-overed, sleazy old goat in the seventies, but I allowed myself to dream. Off around the Colosseum, up through the Botanic Gardens and then I decided to head for home.

I was feeling pretty bloody pleased with myself. The few Romans who were around were bus drivers and early-morning motorists, and despite the fact that I was an overweight 42-year-old with most of my arse hanging out of my running shorts, I'd had a couple of 'Bella, bella!'s and a few wolf whistles. Bless their non-ageist, non-fattist, non-politically correct Latin hearts. They didn't appear to be ironic salutations so I took them in the spirit in which they were intended. The other reason I was feeling fine was that I was starting to feel like a local. I'd visited Rome before a couple of times, and sort of had an idea where the major monuments were, so I decided that I knew my way around.

I was congratulating myself on having such a good sense of location and how surely I must be considered sophisticated to be able to say that I'd jogged around Rome. And that was when I got lost. One ruin looks pretty much like another, and so too does gorgeous beauty. I was running round in circles and although I knew the Pantheon was only minutes away from my hotel, do you think I could work out the right street? I was like a particularly stupid lab rat coming up against brick walls in my maze. As I was running down the Via della Coronia, a good hour after setting out, with no idea where I was or where I was going, I thought how ironic it would be to die of a coronary on the Via della Coronia. Eventually I found a lovely policewoman, all streaked blonde hair and slut-red lipstick, who pointed me in the right direction and I gasped my way back to the hotel foyer, where I collapsed.

I should have known not to be so complacent. Every time I think I'm the remotest bit flash, the Fates conspire to bring me back down to size. When I was 18 and a very junior woodchuck reporter working in Hamilton, my old home town, I was strutting back from an interview with my tape recorder over my shoulder, heading back to the studio. I was kitted out in a skin-tight pencil skirt, my Nova Slides, and a snappy Thornton Hall jacket and as I checked out my reflection in a shop window, I thought I looked quite the business. I sashayed past a huge group of people waiting for buses on Friday afternoon, and thought to myself how they must know I was a girl with a future — it would be obvious to even the most casual passer-by. And with that my Nova Slide high heel got caught in a crack in the pavement, and down I went — right in front of the bus stop crowd. I limped back to the radio station, broken heel, skinned knees, my pride as shattered as the tape recorder and thought to myself that pride really does come before a fall. And ever since that day, no sooner have I thought I might be a cut above the rest, than I'm instantly brought down to size.

There are so many instances, but one other bears mentioning. I was working on the cricket for the Bank of New Zealand years ago — so long ago, that AMI Stadium — Jade Stadium to you traditionalists — was called Lancaster Park. My job was to interview people in the crowd about the day's play and the vox pops, as they're called, would be cut into a one-minute ad, which would screen that night. It was great fun as I love cricket and I was travelling with a great crew. This particular day, we were in Christchurch, and the crowd was riotous. They'd injected watermelon and strawberries with vodka, and that combined with beer and a scorching Canterbury day meant that there were sections of the crowd we didn't dare venture near. I was in a new flirty summer sunfrock and after lunch, I went to the loo and checked myself out in the mirror. I told myself I was holding up very well, and thought how wonderful it was to be me. Young, well, youngish, working with a film crew at the cricket in a pretty dress, getting lots of attention — for a type A personality blonde, life doesn't really get much better. The crew were waiting for me at the far end of the ground, so I made my way towards them. The cheers and hoots of appreciation were enormously gratifying. The crowd was going wild — I tuned out the actual words and just revelled in the attention. I slowed down my walk, pushed my boobs out and swung my hips —

I was working that crowd, baby. Tyra Banks had nothing on me. As I neared the crew, one of the girls said: What on earth was all that about? Oh, I said, tossing my head, walking past her, and resting my elbows on the ground railing, looking nonchalantly out to the middle where the cricket was about to resume, I have no idea. Um, I think I do, said the soundman. Your dress is tucked up right into the back of your G-string. So yes. I'm now very wary of ever thinking life is too sweet and I blame my lapse in Rome on jetlag.

After a couple of days in Rome, our party boarded the *Wind Surf*, the beautiful yacht we were to spend the next ten days aboard. She was exquisite and although she was small, there was indeed a gym, as promised. I planned an hour's run on the machine every day, and when I announced my intention, my Irishman managed not to scoff and said that would be a great effort. Of course, he knew and I knew there'd be nothing of the kind. I managed just the one. But I suppose all the walking we did, around Amalfi and Taormina and Dubrovnik mitigated against the lack of running. It wouldn't have mitigated against the copious amounts of food and booze I was chucking down my throat, but hey, what's a girl to do? How much fun would I have been for the rest of the group if I'd been a lentil-munching wowser? Oh, yes. Runners' justifications and excuses. I've heard and uttered them all.

After the cruise, which was simply fabulous, we had a week in a villa in Florence. The villa was absolutely gorgeous — just down the road from San Gimignano, right in the heart of Tuscany. However, it appeared to be a type of retreat for young executives and honeymooning couples.

Fresh-faced, fit young things wandered around the place in white hooded robes, speaking in hushed tones, ordering mineral water and freshly squeezed juices. Either that or we'd stumbled on a weird religious cult. I half-expected to see Tom Cruise draped across a lounger by the pool. A bunch of thirty raucous Kiwis crashing about the place somewhat shattered the ambience, but the good part about it being a health spa was that there was a gym tucked away in the basement. I dragged myself away from the pool and the shopping and one afternoon I managed a run on the machine. A couple of the boys from my tour group came down to witness with their very own eyes the fact that I could actually run. They stood in the doorway as I tried to run and talk and not trip over my feet and then wandered away to have a beer. Which would have been much more fun for them than watching me bouncing up and down. But there it was. One one-hour run. I also managed a massage. On a very cool table. The spa had waterbed-type massage tables so you just sort of sank into them when the softly spoken girls with muscular triceps pushed and rubbed. Very nice. But not exactly conducive to running a marathon. And then I was home.

Things were starting to get a bit desperate. It was two months to the New York Marathon and I needed to get some good long runs under my belt. In fact, any runs at all would have done. I was managing about three a week, nowhere near as many as I'd been doing before Auckland, and I was starting to have grave fears about my ability to run the bloody thing. I knew I would finish — if needs be, I'd just walk — and that's the advantage of having done one before. It's the fear of the unknown that really paralyses

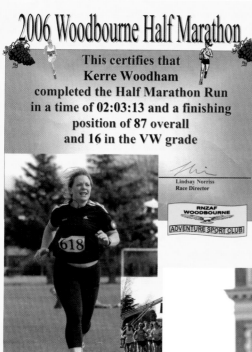

Look at the size of my gut! The photo that nearly caused me to give up the whole enterprise.

2006 Woodbourne Half Marathon

This certifies that
Kerre Woodham
completed the Half Marathon Run
in a time of **02:03:13** and a finishing
position of 87 overall
and 16 in the VW grade

Lindsay Norriss
Race Director

RNZAF
WOODBOURNE
ADVENTURE SPORT CLUB

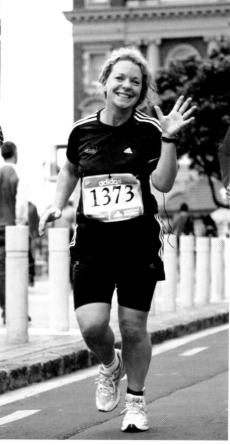

The adidas Auckland Marathon — on the home straight, feeling good, just one k to go.

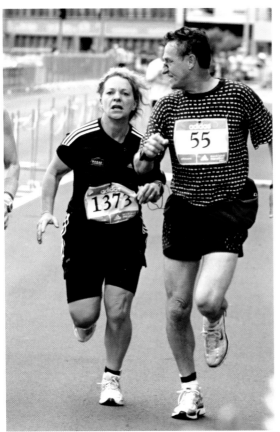

My running mate, Bruce, was determined we'd make it home in under 4:30. With just metres to go, Bruce is telling me to put my head down and run.

Seconds to go till the end of my first marathon. Clearly there's no such thing as a typical marathon runner.

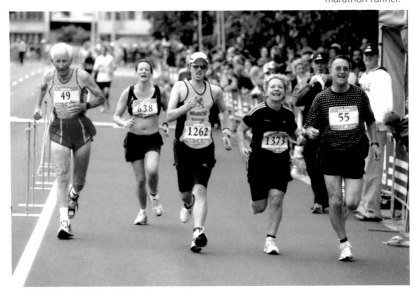

I did it! Pure and utter elation at crossing the line — alive and in one piece.

Photo by Richard Robinson, courtesy *New Zealand Herald*.

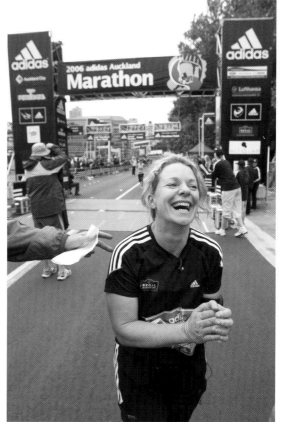

The reason for running — handing over the $5000 cheque to Alex Powell, Auckland president of the Cystic Fibrosis Association, and her gorgeous daughter, Bella.

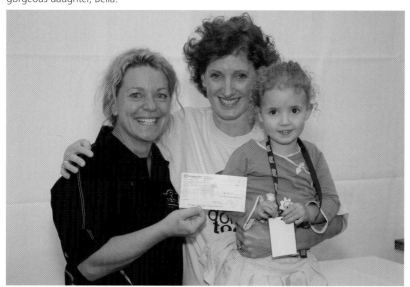

My trainer, Gaz. Couldn't have done it without him.

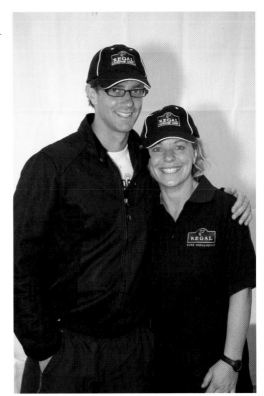

At the Rachel Hunter fundraiser for Breast Cancer. I didn't let social events interfere with my training — I was up at 7 a.m. for the Saturday morning run; my New York team-mate Blair (second from left), however, didn't make it.

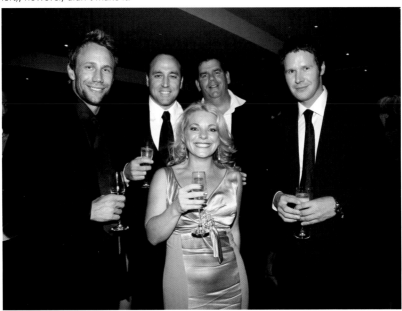

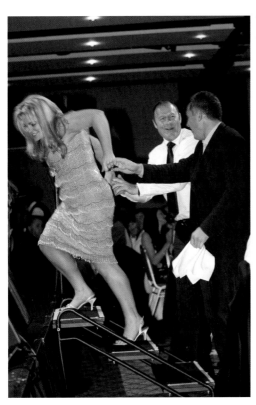

Weight training with former All Blacks Alan Whetton and Frank Bunce — I was speaking at Tana Umaga's celebrity roast.

Picking up our race numbers in New York — the excitement is clear! Left to right, back row: Jean-Michel, Hilary, our illustrious leader Gaz, me, Geeling; front row: Kamilla, Steven, Livvy.

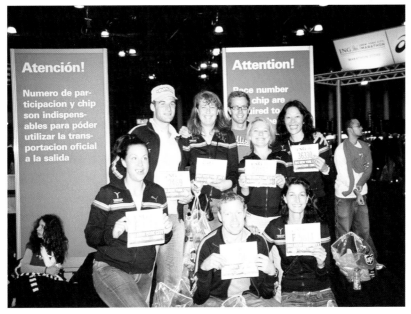

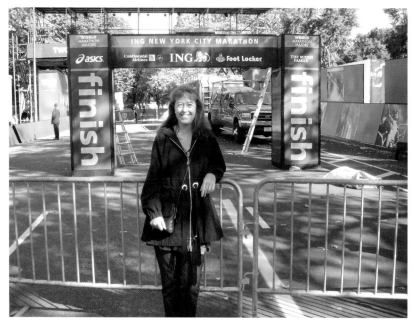

Hils visualising the finish — Central Park, New York.

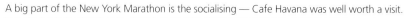

A big part of the New York Marathon is the socialising — Cafe Havana was well worth a visit.

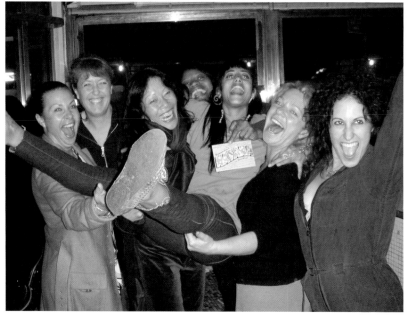

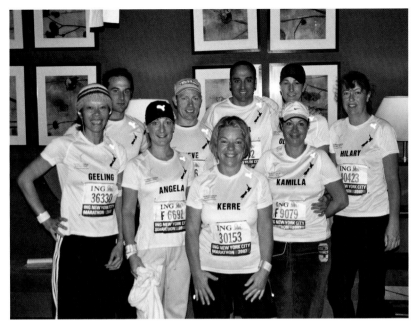

The day of reckoning — 5.30 a.m. in our hotel lobby, about to set off.

Lachie leading the support team — what would we have done without our support crew?

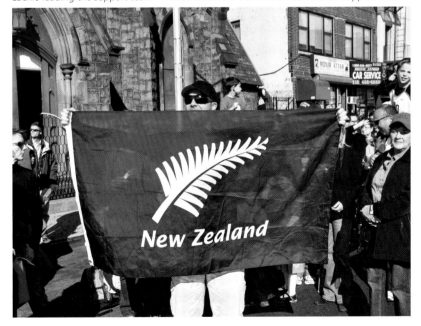

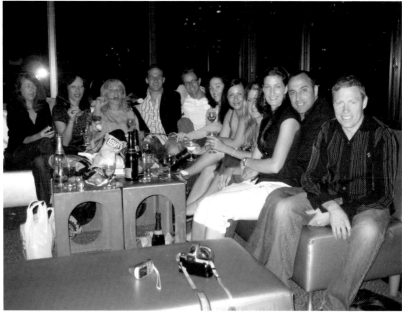

Enjoying a celebratory drink just a few hours after the New York Marathon.

Eat your heart out, Katie Holmes! Out clubbing the night of the marathon — our heels were higher, our boys were hotter, we stayed out longer.

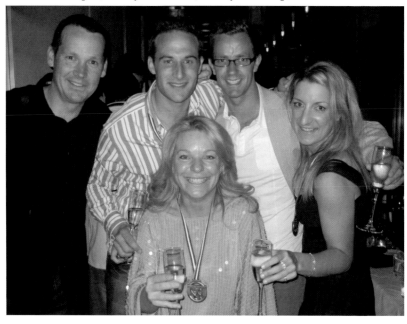

people. If you know what you're in for, then at least you can plan. But I wanted to have a good time. The Mission: Possible team was a great group of people and I didn't want to be in such a bad state when I finished that I wouldn't be able to enjoy the Big Apple in their company. So it was time to go to work.

I wasn't able to run the with Rats, as every Friday night I had black tie functions to MC as I had to pay my way to New York. Prancing around on stage, commanding and maintaining the attention of hundreds of people takes it out of a girl. On bad nights, when I've wondered how I'm going to capture an inebriated audience, hours after I get home I'm still shaking from the adrenalin and nerves and sheer energy it takes to get people to sit still, listen to me and laugh. Apparently, the shock to your system when you're public speaking is equivalent to the shock you suffer in a non-injury car crash — on that basis, I was crashing every weekend! Consequently, I was too knackered to get up in the morning at 6 a.m. to head out to Titters for my long run, and although the Mission:Possible team started their runs later in the day, it wasn't much point going with them, as most of them were younger, stronger and faster and I'd end up running at my own pace anyway, so I might as well run from home. Mary, Lavina and Lee weren't available to run with me this year as Mary had switched to a new challenge and was training for the Round Taupo cycle race and Lavina was pregnant with her third beautiful baby. Lee, too, found out she was pregnant just after completing the New York Marathon, in defiance of all medical odds. There you go. Having trouble getting pregnant? Run a marathon. So my usual suspects weren't available and my own erratic timetable meant I wasn't a good enough bet to hook up with a new training partner. Running on my own meant the runs were shorter and less intense and I didn't feel the same pressure to get out the door when I didn't have a couple of runners waiting on the corner for me. I was on my own and that made it tough.

There was one memorable Saturday when I was just heading out to join my team-mates for a rare Saturday morning excursion. I literally had one foot out the door, I was in my gear, Vaseline on all my delicate bits, when my cellphone rang. I was going to ignore it and then I thought it might be one of the team looking for a lift down to the waterfront, so I went back into my room and picked it up. It wasn't a number I recognised, but I answered it anyway — it must be important if someone was ringing at 7 a.m. on a Saturday — and by crikey, it was. It was Olivia from the Child Cancer Foundation wanting to know if I wanted a lift out to the Waipuna Hotel where I was to be speaking to the mums of kids with cancer at their conference breakfast.

'Today?' I gasped. 'This morning?'

'Yes,' she replied nervously. 'You did remember, didn't you?'

'I thought it was next weekend,' I stammered. 'Hang on, I'll be there in a tick. What time does it start?'

'Eight,' she replied. 'It will be a shame if you can't make it. They're expecting you.' The disappointed reproach was obvious in her tone.

I hung up, raced into the shower, washed off the Vaseline, and buried my face in a bucket of foundation on the way out the door. I was chilled to the bone with horror at the thought I might have forgotten. Imagine letting down the parents of children with cancer! What sort of low-life would do that? Imagine if Olivia had rung me just a minute later: I'd have been in the car, on my way to the waterfront, running jauntily round the Viaduct with not a care in the world while back at the Waipuna Hotel, a room full of mums with horribly sick children, waited. It just didn't bear thinking about.

Still, I got out to the hotel just in time, and was introduced to Louise. Louise would be introducing me to the room. She was a lovely woman, living in Gisborne, whose wee boy had been diagnosed with cancer and, after a long battle, looked like he'd come through. She stood up and began to speak and I realised that this Louise was the same Louise who, several months earlier, had emailed me at the radio station to find out how to go about entering the New York Marathon. She was unable to get television where she lived so had been forced to become a talkback listener and had followed my progress through my marathon training and the subsequent decision to enter New York and decided she'd give it a go too. I'd put her in touch with Carole Mills from Travel Managers Group and we'd exchanged a few emails since. She'd been training on her own, around the hill country of the remote sheep station where she lived with her husband and two children, and she wanted to run the marathon to celebrate her fortieth birthday. It was wonderful to put a gorgeous face to a name, and yet another reason why I was so very glad I'd had the phone call from Olivia.

I came home, thoroughly shaken. I had a lot of work on, there was a lot of training to do, and I simply couldn't afford to be so disorganised. I had the best of intentions to buy myself a Blackberry (and learn how to use it); to use the calendar on my computer; hell, I didn't even have to really use technology. I could just write in the dates of engagements in pen on my wall calendar! But just as I have always written essays and newspaper columns (and books!) at the last minute, pushing right up to deadlines and beyond, I thrive on pressure and I just had to accept that that was my nature and while I could try to be switched on and diligent, I would probably fail.

And so the half-hearted, desultory training continued. I managed a two-and-a-half hour run in the wind and rain round the waterfront and back, building up to the team 33 km run which was taking place on Labour Weekend. My solo run nearly ended in disaster as I'd diligently wrapped lambswool around my toes to protect against blistering. About 10 km in, I stopped at the public loos and used a piece of the wool to stop the chafing of my wet bra under my boobs. It worked a treat and I was feeling quite proud of myself for being so innovative — and there it was again. Pride coming before a fall. I became aware that the ache in my toe was not the usual sort of ache I was used to. I soldiered on for a while, telling myself not to be so pathetic and reminding myself that I was looking for any excuse to give up and walk for a while, when I decided that before I pushed on the last 6 km to home, I should check to make sure there was nothing seriously wrong. I pulled off my shoe and sock, and just as well I did, as when I'd rewrapped the wool around my toes, I'd wrapped it far too tightly around my second toe. It had been deprived of blood for about an hour and subjected to intolerable pressure and was about to drop off. Well, not really. I exaggerate. But it was certainly a very unhealthy blue colour. I grappled at the wet wool, which had formed itself almost into a tight plaster cast and eventually managed to get it off and home I jogged, with no real harm done. I pulled up OK after that run and my foot hadn't given me any major problems — other than when I'd applied a toe tourniquet — so that was an encouraging sign. Once you run a marathon, maybe you reach a certain base level of fitness that never leaves you, no matter how lazy you are. I was hoping, anyway.

The last payment had been made for New York and the departure date was looming. Eight-tenths of the Mission: Possible team was able to gather together for a team run — the long run — before we began our taper. The taper is a rest period before the marathon and is just as important as the training itself, but Gaz will tell you all about that. I'd been tapering all bloody year, so it wasn't as important for me. But some of the others were training hard and needed that rest time if they weren't going to injure themselves. We all gathered at one of the cafés near the Viaduct and set off on the route that Gaz had devised. Some of the runners Gaz was training for the Auckland Marathon also came with us, and a couple of volunteers from the Breast Cancer Research Trust, the charity we were running for, came along to hand out water, lollies and encouragement along the way, which was jolly decent of them. Even more impressive, however, was the appearance of one of our number, Blair, who turned up on his mountain bike. Since the team had gathered together back in late January, I had seen Blair just the once. And that was at a black tie charity do where neither of us was running — except to the bar. He'd told us all right from the start that Saturday morning runs were damn near impossible and he doubted he would make it. He was right. Our 40-something party boy failed to show at any of the runs, but it was impressive to see him make it for the big one. Even if it was on his bike. This time, he had a legitimate reason for not running — he needed to give shin splints time to recover — but the fact that he'd turned up to support his fellow team members cheered us all. Gaz finally showed up to get us under way — it had been his birthday the night before and he was a little under the weather — and then we were off, with the good runners setting off like hares and the little round tortoises, Kamilla and me, bringing up the rear.

It was great having Kamilla to run with, but at the 12 km mark she told me to run on ahead. And I did. I love having someone to run with, but I much prefer running at my own pace. Up we wound through the streets of St Heliers and Glen Innes — and suddenly there were two of the front runners, belting along heading for home before I'd even hit the turn. Jean-Michel and Steven were going to do very good times in New York and they were looking in great shape. JM asked me if I needed any water — he had some spares — and offered words of encouragement without slowing his pace. I was fine and wished him well and told him I'd see him — eventually — back at the café. Which I did. Slowly, steadily and buoyed by the occasional appearances of Gaz, Blair and Helen, one of the Auckland runners, I made it back to base without having a cardiac infarction. I was pleased that my foot seemed to have come right, and delighted that I'd got the long run out of the way. I hadn't been able to do one before Auckland, and that had caused me great angst and consternation. Now, however, I'd done it and was completely confident I'd take New York.

The other runners had finished quite some time before me so we waited a while for Kamilla before deciding to head into the café to wait for her there. We'd just started on our first lattes when in she came. Well stuff that, she announced in a loud voice to the room at large. She looked utterly fed up and it seemed to be more than just the natural exhaustion you feel after a long run. What's up? we asked.

'I decided,' she said, plonking herself down in a chair, 'to take a short cut through the Viaduct because I'd been out there for hours and I'd had enough.'

We all murmured soothing words of support and she went on.

'And so I was running past all the bars and cafés — which, of course, were full because it's Labour Weekend, and everyone in Auckland was out having brunch — and this smelly old wino was sitting on a park bench. He called out to me, "Jeez. You looked stuffed." And I said to him, I *am* stuffed. I've been running for four hours. "Four hours?" he said incredulously. "Have you? Then how come your arse is still so big?" '

We all shrieked. Kamilla's got a great sense of humour and she could see the funny side of it. To make matters worse, the wino called out to all the Saturday café set — Check her out! She's been running for four hours and her arse is wobbling. Kamilla tried to clench and run, almost pulling a hammy, and made it back to the sanctity of the group. Oh, Kamilla, I said when I could finally stop laughing. That story's going in the book. And it has.

My mum was up staying for the long weekend, and I'd promised her that Kate and I would take her shopping once I'd got the run out of the way. I came home to find my wonderful Irishman had run the bath for me, and I had a languorous soak before heading out again. I have a special expensive body scrub with a delicious smell that I reward myself with after long runs, so I scrubbed the sweat and the city grime off myself and headed out, fragrant and well pleased with my morning's work. The three of us wandered along the streets and Mum headed into Kumfs, a store I'd always thought of as a shoe shop for oldies who can't handle wearing high heels. Mum decided to try on a pair of shoes, which really were very nice and pretty snazzy for a seventy-year-old, and I spotted some flat shoes that would be perfect for wearing with jeans. Try them on, Mum urged, and the moment I did I was sold. My poor abused feet collapsed into them and it felt like I was walking on air. I bought them on the spot and walked out in them, and I don't care that I've crossed that line. Once you become a Kumfs wearer, that's it, really. You're on the downward slide. But if you're a marathon runner, your poor feet deserve a break. No matter what your age, get yourself along to your local Kumfs store or something similar, put aside any pretensions and prejudices and treat your feet. They'll love you for it.

We had just over a week to go before we headed off to New York and we had a champagne breakfast planned to raise money for the BCRT and act as a thank you to our friends, families and supporters. Being the resident rent-a-mouth, I was MCing, but Livvy, the long-legged lovely of our group, had done a magnificent job getting together fabulous auction items and chivvying along people to come to the event. She and Gaz were phenomenal in generating sponsorship and publicity and they really were the driving force of the fundraising. It was a stellar success, raising about $12,000, and was a fitting send-off for the team. The next day, the Sunday, was the day of the Auckland Marathon, and although I dearly wanted to cheer on the Auckland runners, I work on Sunday mornings on the radio and I'd taken so much time off work with my trip to Europe and the forthcoming trip to New York, it was impossible. However, I caught up with two of my Auckland running friends, Helen and Tina, at the home of their trainer and it was wonderful hearing their war stories and seeing the absolute thrill of achievement on their faces. Once you've run a marathon, that's it. You will forever more be a marathon runner and no-one can take that away from you. You are one of a rare and special breed that has had the grit, the determination and the bloodymindedness to train for six months to endure one of the toughest tests anyone can put their body through. The girls were proud of themselves and they had every right to be so.

GAZ

I find my hardest job is fitting a structured and consistent running programme into an average person's busy life. There's always a holiday planned for the year and it's usually at least two weeks long. On average you can get away with two weeks without training, but after that you lose your fitness dramatically, and it can take twice as long to get it back. I like to put people on maintenance programmes while they are on vacation. These are designed to maintain your current fitness level, but they will not get you any quicker or stronger. You have to be realistic; after all, when you're on holiday you should be enjoying yourself, not putting yourself through the mill. I recommend that my runners try to complete three runs per week while on holiday. They don't have to be long; a half hour on each run will suffice, as long as they are completed.

Another aspect I always have to take into consideration is that people have social lives. I don't like to train my clients by ruling with an iron fist, it's just not my style. Don't get me wrong, if the training is not being completed, then a word has to be said, but I think there should be a balance, although in Kerre's case the balance is usually a little towards the social side! Some alcohol is fine — it's been proven that a glass or two wine a day can be beneficial to health. Just remember, that's two glasses and not two fishbowls, as in the Mission: Possible team's case! At least you're a cheap drunk when you're a runner, as your tolerance for alcohol becomes a lot lower.

The long run is considered the most important part of your training programme. This is when you get an idea of what it is going to feel like on the day. Although your long run may not be as long as the marathon itself, coupled with the kilometres you have completed that week it will bring you very close to the feeling, just minus the euphoria. It's the one time that you get to really see what your body is capable of. It seems amazing that you can start off running 10 minutes and a year later — or less — be running for a whole 32 km. It's a chance to sit back and realise just how far you have come. Too often we get caught up in what we haven't done and forget to look back and soak up what we have achieved. The great thing about finishing a truly long run is the surge of endorphins that releases. These are natural feel-good hormones, the cause of the 'runner's high'. If you ask me, there's no better sensation than finishing a run and getting that endorphin release. It's better than any magic pill and a damn sight better for you!

I try to have each beginner-level client complete three long runs before they tackle a marathon. These are usually 28 km, 30 km and 32 km, although I tweak that depending on the ability of the individual. What you will find critical is the rest between these runs. This is the time when it becomes crucial to really read your body and listen to any signals it is giving you. These long runs are important. You have to do whatever you can to prepare for them. That means that you don't go out on a bender the night before a long run (unless it's your birthday) and you get as much sleep as possible.

You may find that you have to change your planned running schedule between these long runs. That's why it's a great idea to have a coach (of course, www.getrunning.co.nz, Gaz Brown Personal Training is the preferred option here!). Depending on how well a person pulls up from their long run, I might remove or reduce a couple sessions in the week leading up to the next long run. You should come into that next run feeling fresh, and if that means you only get two runs in, then so be it. Just make sure you replace the other sessions with an alternative like swimming or cycling. Finally, make sure you have a great support crew out on the run. There's nothing better than seeing someone sitting on the corner waiting for you with an abundance of power gels, food and drink. It gives you that feeling of accomplishment and lets you know that it really is all about you!

The tapering section of the programme is the time when

you start to feel great. Up to this stage your body will have been stressed then rested, stressed then rested and so on. Just when you feel like you are getting stronger, the programme steps up another notch! It's not until you come into the taper weeks that you realise how fit you really are. You'll be able to jump buildings in single bounds and climb walls! Well, at least for some! Often I have seen runners' bodies pretty stressed by this stage and the taper phase allows their bodies to get rid of all those little niggles before the big day. There is a fine line between a taper and too much rest, though, and you have to ensure that you keep your body ready for the big day. This is not the time to catch up on the social life that you lost three months before!

chapter nine

New York, New York

And then, all of a sudden, it was Tuesday and we were packed and ready to go. Because of stuffing around on the airline's part, we had to catch an obscenely early flight to Sydney to catch a connecting flight to Los Angeles to catch a connecting flight to New York. It was going to be a marathon just getting there. And so it proved to be. It was Kamilla's birthday and she was going to have it in three different countries in three different time zones. Gaz had arranged lounge passes for all of us in Sydney as a surprise, so we toasted Kamilla with champagne and then had a bit more, just for good measure. We were part of a bigger group of Kiwis travelling over for the marathon, but it wasn't till we got to New York, about twenty-six hours later, that we all met one another as we boarded the bus. We were part of the Travel Managers group, led by Carole Mills, but it wasn't an escorted tour as such. We were all just runners and walkers who'd paid our way into the marathon. Many of the participants had come over as individuals and some had come with their adult children to fulfil a dream together, which was inspirational. I was glad I was part of a team. Some of our members had brought their partners over, but there were still about seven of us who could play together. It made it so much more fun.

I'd been to New York before, back in 2000, when I was filming a television show I won't mention because it sank like a stone and you won't have heard of it. The hotel the crew and I had stayed in was right on Central Park, but I remembered the room as being absolutely tiny and having no windows. I'd arrived from Paris, taken one look at my room, and marched down to reception to talk to the manager.

'My room doesn't appear to have any windows,' I said nicely. 'It's a little claustrophobic. Is it possible to change? I'm quite happy to pay more.'

The manager didn't even look up from the girlie mag he was reading.

'You don' like it — check out,' he spat.

Quite literally. Out of the corner of his mouth into what I hoped was a spittoon at his feet. I scuttled back upstairs and resolved to put up with my airless cell — and the dead body from the room next door that paramedics were removing as I unpacked my not-so smalls into the veneer wood drawers. The body went, but the NYPD tape across the door stayed for the duration of our residency.

So my memories of New York hotels were not that great. However, Carole had done a great job sourcing our hotel. It was on the East Side, overlooking the East River. I had a room on my own, and it was absolutely enormous, with floor-to-ceiling windows that afforded a view over the river as well as the street. It was so exciting to be back in New York. I felt so privileged that I'd had the good fortune to have the resources, the family and the job that allowed me time away to fulfil another personal goal. It had been a real drag getting to this point. I was fighting myself every inch of the way. There were many, many occasions when I had felt like throwing in the towel, but I hadn't and now here I was. About to run the New York Marathon, along with 39,999 people from all around the globe. Actually, I think it was only because we were paying as we went that I continued to train for the marathon. Had we just had to pay one lump payment a couple of weeks before we left, I think I would have probably pulled out. However, having committed a couple of thousand dollars towards the trip, I had to keep going. I wonder if Carole plans the payments that way — to help maintain people's motivation!

We bunked down for the night, and rose bright and early to head down and get our registration packs. We all wore our BCRT jackets and there was a real sense of adventure walking down to Grand Central Station, where we'd take the bus to the Expo Centre. Hilary, who'd joined us from Paris, had already worked out the best way to get to the station, so we followed her lead, committing to memory Bloomingdales and Saks 5th Avenue and the Ed Hardy store and all the fabulous shops we intended to come back to visit. It felt like a school outing with only the very coolest kids. We had no idea how to get where we were going, but New Yorkers were incredibly friendly and helpful when they knew we were here for the marathon. This first-day friendliness was indicative of the attitude of the whole city. They were never too busy to help us out, and everyone we spoke to enjoyed the same experience. Obviously, the huge number of runners brings an economic boost to the city, but the friendliness went beyond that: the American attitude of celebrating individual achievement meant they were delighted to support us, in whatever way they could, in attaining our goal.

The registration process went like clockwork. There were hundreds of volunteers on hand, ensuring we all had our race-day bags within twenty minutes of walking through the door. It was an amazing feeling getting our race numbers and our T-shirts. It was really hitting home now, and the warm welcome we received from the men and women manning the desks made us feel like we were truly a part of something special. Most of our team decided to have a look around all the sports shoes and running gear for sale, but Geeling and I decided to head back to town and have a look around the city. She's been to New York a few times and has very well-connected friends, so she had a fair idea where all the hot and trendy restaurants were. As you can imagine, I was quite happy to tag along with Gee wherever she wanted to go.

We got the bus as far into town as it would take us and began walking back to the hotel when we passed a sign saying The Russian Tea Rooms. Do you think it's *the* Russian Tea Rooms, asked Geeling. We'd both heard of the famous restaurant established by White Russians fleeing the Communists nearly a hundred years ago, but America is the land of the franchise. There could have been hundreds of them dotted throughout the city. However, the doorman, resplendent in top hat and tails, assured us that this was indeed the one and only and Geeling and I walked through the revolving door and into red velvet opulence. Priceless art works hung on the walls and all around us people sat in red leather banquettes sipping champagne. Geeling and I were still in our jeans and BCRT jackets, but the suave mâitre d' assured us we were perfectly adequately dressed and ushered us to a table. It was simply splendid. Pink champagne and a caviar omelette. The perfect lunch for a marathon runner. The mâitre d' was delightful and after we'd finished lunch he showed us around the three floors of the restaurant. It's absolutely beautiful and well worth checking out if you make it over to New York — the highlight being a dancing bear, made out of glass, filled with goldfish, on the second floor! Geeling and I were suitably appreciative and after our tour, we left amidst many protestations of goodwill. Gee and I parted company and I wandered back to the hotel, soaking up the sights and the sounds.

This set the pattern for our time in New York. There was always someone around if you wanted company, and if you didn't, well, that was just fine too. A hard-core group of six or seven of us generally met up for dinner and it was wonderful getting to know everyone better over beautiful food and great wine. Probably if we were aiming for world-record times we would have steered clear of the booze, but we weren't. The majority of us were sloggers hoping to finish and the fast runners were young enough and confident enough to assume that a couple of glasses of wine wouldn't make a difference. We shopped up a storm, visited museums, drank far too much and laughed almost constantly. I wasn't getting much sleep — the jet lag I experienced in New York was worse than anything

I'd ever suffered in Europe and I found myself waking at 1 and 4 a.m. every morning. It was infuriating, but then I didn't have any responsibilities in New York. No dog to walk, meals to cook, house to clean or talkback callers to attract. The only downside was not having the Irishman or Kate with me. I would have loved to have shared the experience of New York with the two people I love most in the world, but being on my own, and yet part of the team, was the second best thing.

The Friendship Run is a short jog for runners who've come from all points of the globe to participate in the New York Marathon. It's run the day before the marathon proper, and generally attracts tens of thousands of runners looking to shake out their legs before the big day. It begins outside the United Nations building on 1st and 44th, and is about 3 km long, ending up on 6th and 54th. To be perfectly honest, on the Saturday morning I would have preferred a sleep-in. A group of us had taken the bus out to Woodbury Common, a shopping village an hour from New York City and is a designer outlet paradise. On the plane over, I found myself next to a good-looking young Irishman based in Australia, who spent a lot of time in New York. He told me about Woodbury Common and insisted it was well worth the trip out. I was somewhat dubious. In my experience, discount and designer outlets usually mean missing sequins and tatty rubbish, but he was well dressed and impeccably groomed, so Kamilla, Gaz, JM and I decided it was worth a look. And, oh my God! You have to see it to believe it. We sacrificed ourselves on the altar of commerce and only stopped when we ran out of funds. The boys in particular discovered their inner shoppers and unleashed them with a vengeance. On the bus home, they could barely contain themselves with the excitement of scoring truly stupendous bargains. G-Star jeans for $5; Hugo Boss jackets for a hundy; Calvin Klein boxers for a fiver — we sat in the back of the bus oohing and aahing over one another's purchases and were so pleased with ourselves that we decided to revisit the Russian Tea Rooms and celebrate our good fortune with some restorative glasses of champagne. Hell, we'd saved so much money we could afford to. Which is a particularly feminine logic, I know, but the boys were so suffused with oestrogen after their day's shopping that they agreed. Hilary met us there and a glass of champagne turned into rather more than was strictly wise for a group of marathon runners, but the pizza from the pizzeria across the road soaked it up. And the red wine we consumed with the pizza is known to be a good anti-oxidant.

What with all the excitement, however, and the fact that I was still waking up at 1 and at 4, regular as clockwork, when the phone rang and Gaz ordered me to get my sorry ass down to the foyer for the Friendship Run, I didn't feel particularly disposed to be friendly to anyone. And I certainly didn't feel like running. It was cold, too, and there were literally thousands of people jostling for position inside the grounds of the United Nations building. Each country had a flag bearer — ours was a runner trying to qualify for the Beijing Olympics, but being 5 foot 1 and a half — don't forget the half — I missed most of the ceremony. I feel like an oversized dog in crowds — I'm so short my view is restricted to crotches and armpits and I rely on people relaying information to know what's going on. The ceremony itself I found boring, but if you're tall you might get a kick out of it. The run, however, was cool. Running down 6th Avenue, knowing that the roads in one of the world's busiest cities have been blocked off just for you, is a fabulous feeling. We all ran together and spent most of the time gazing around us in wonder and repeating to one another just how amazing this all was and how very lucky we were to be here.

After the run we walked back to the diner near our hotel and had a whopper of an American breakfast. Brilliant breakfasts in New York, except they cannot make a decent cup of coffee to save their lives. If I was young, I'd be over there in a flash, with a couple of hot baristas in tow. Kerre's Klassic Koffees would have made an absolute fortune. Minor gripe, however. I wandered up the road to the hairdresser and booked in to get my hair washed and blow waved after the marathon. I've never been able to do my own hair. Left to itself it looks like a particularly frizzy pubic mound, so I put it in the hands of experts if I'm going somewhere special. And as we'd planned to paint the town vermilion after our run, I needed my hair looking good. The girls at the salon were lovely and I made an appointment for three. However, back at the hotel, I did some mental arithmetic. Yes, we were getting up at 4 a.m. the next morning to run the marathon, but it didn't actually start until 10 a.m. There was every chance I'd still be running at 3 o'clock! And I still had to get back to the hotel. I rang the girls and they agreed to shift the appointment to five. Surely I'd have finished running by then.

Gaz delivered our T-shirts to us — Puma had kindly

sponsored them — and Gaz had had them printed with a little map of New Zealand, the Breast Cancer Research Trust logo and our names. Everyone who runs the New York Marathon needs to get their name printed on their shirts as the crowd will call out your name and encourage you on personally, which makes the occasion much more special than an all-purpose 'You go, girl!' I had forgotten to suggest to Gaz that he misspell my name, as Kerre is an unorthodox spelling, and I didn't really want to run 42 km with a whole bunch of well-meaning New Yorkers yelling what sounded like 'Go, Cur!' However, I'd forgotten and there it was — Kerre emblazoned across my chest. I set out everything I'd need for the next day — my shorts, my leggings, my barrier cream, bra, wool for my toes, socks, shoes, shirt, twenty bucks for catching a cab home afterwards and a couple of sticking plasters. The rest of the day was spent trying to relax and prepare myself for the big day. And trying to put the death of a young US marathoner out of my mind.

Earlier that morning, as the Friendship Run was taking place, the US Olympic men's marathon trial was being run in Central Park. Five miles in, one of the top runners, 28-year-old Ryan Shay, collapsed and died.

He was as fit as a buck rat but he was unable to be revived and was pronounced dead on arrival at Lennox Hospital. There seemed to be no rhyme nor reason for his death and it was a sobering news story — literally and metaphorically. If a fit young élite athlete like that could die during a marathon, what hope did an overweight old tart have, especially when she hadn't given the marathon the respect it deserved. I tried to put the story to one side and concentrate on positive thinking, but I'm sure the news of Ryan Shay's death was a shock for many of us who were due to line up at the start line in twenty-four hours.

We'd booked in for a pasta dinner at an Italian restaurant up the road, and it was a time for us all to bond. However, the manager had massively overbooked — there were 39,980 other runners and their supporters who were all turning up at Italian restaurants to carbo load too — so we had to wait for about forty minutes. Some people were getting a little edgy as they had a strict routine they were following and wanted to make sure they got a good night's sleep, but finally the mâitre d' seated us, and made up for the delay by giving us all good luck charms for the race the next day. Traditionally, there is a pasta meal up at the Tavern on the Green in Central Park, but you get a ticket, you sit at a bench table, you scarf it down and then you're moved on. Didn't sound like much fun to me, and besides, we were in New York, the home of great food. Why would you eat crap when you could eat something fabulous? But I would recommend you make a booking at an Italian restaurant close to where you're staying before you even leave New Zealand, otherwise you may find yourself eating at Subway or the local Pizza Hutt and that would be a shame.

It was the night before, and I lay in my huge bed, looking at the beautiful flowers my Irishman had sent from New Zealand to wish me luck. There were lovely messages of support and encouragement that had been emailed to me as well, but I was feeling ambivalent about the run. Although I'd done the long run and had pulled up fine after it, really, I hadn't done enough training. I was carrying about 4 kilos more into this marathon than I had into Auckland and when you're running 42 km, every little gram counts. I'd done a marathon before, so I didn't feel the same sick excitement I'd felt last year, when I didn't know what my body could do. On the plus side, I was in New York! I was going to run the New York Marathon! And that counted for a lot.

I hate getting up in the morning. I've already mentioned how concerned I was about getting up early for the Auckland Marathon, but there was no getting away from a dawn rising in New York. Other members of the Kiwi team running and walking the marathon headed off at 4 a.m., but Gaz decided — and we members of Team Mission: Possible agreed — that if we were in the lobby at 5.15, that would give us enough time to get from our hotel to the library, where buses would ferry us across to Staten Island and the marathon start line. Although I'd been waking all week at 4 a.m., sod's law says I would sleep in on the very morning I needed to be awake bright and early, so it was a phone call from Gaz that got me out of bed. I threw on my clothes and tore down to the lobby, terrified that I was either keeping the others waiting or that they'd left without me. Fortunately for me, Hils and Livvy had also slept in, so I wasn't the last one down.

Nick had already left — he didn't want to be in any way stressed and wanted to have plenty of time up his sleeve, so it was just the nine of us to make our way across town to the library. There was hardly anyone on the streets, which put the wind up us a bit. Surely we hadn't left it too late. And it seemed a whole lot further than we'd been told. The twenty-minute walk was more like a forty-minute walk, which seemed a bit unnecessary given that we were going to be running 42 km later in the day. Eventually we turned the corner and saw a long line of buses and people in runners clothes being herded onto them efficiently and smoothly. New York has got people management down to a fine art. We walked straight onto a bus and then we were off, like kids on a school trip, laughing and chatting excitedly. There was a moment of silence as we crossed the Staten Bridge and looked back towards the city and the enormity of what we were about to undertake hit home. But then we were back into it again, and we disembarked at Fort Wadsworth, once one of the United States' most important military installations. It's now under the guardianship of the National Park Service and home to the Coastguard and this is where we were to wait for the start gun.

Obviously, with 40,000 people, the start times were staggered. The good runners, the ones running for money, people like world record holder Paula Radcliffe, would go first, unimpeded by weekend plodders like me. And then the rest of us came about forty minutes later. We were grouped in colours and each colour group went off at a different time, but the groupings seemed to defy any sort of logic. I was in the same group as JM and Steven — the two fastest runners in our team. Explain that one! Still, I was grateful that I had some of my team members with me. It would have been a lonely experience waiting nearly three hours to start without a mate there with you. Old pros at the New York Marathon game had brought old deck chairs, lilos and inflatable rings to sit on and read the paper — I'd thought about doing something along those lines, but again, putting the thought into action is often where I stumble. There were water stations, Dunkin Donut bagels, free Gatorade and first-aid tents within every holding area and, of course, there were the inevitable queues for the Portaloos.

Steven, JM and I found a spot to sit, munched on bagels and bided our time. The wait until the start went quite quickly. We were lucky that it was perfect marathon-running weather — cool, clear and sunny. I can't imagine what it would have been like waiting three and a half hours in driving wind, rain or snow. You're totally exposed to the elements and the weather is notoriously unpredictable. It's a good idea to bear in mind that you could be running in any sort of conditions, so bring along a range of suitable clothing that you're prepared to dump on the start line. I wore an old pair of track pants and an old jacket, which I chucked once we started heading for the line. I didn't bother checking in a bag. The queues for the UPS trucks were worse than those for the Portaloos and I wanted to make a quick getaway at the end. The thought of queuing for my bag in Central Park at the end of a torturous run didn't do it for me at all. However, the others were happy to drop their bags, so I left them to it and made my way to the part of our staging area where the pace-setters were gathered.

I was trying for a 4:30 marathon — I realised it was wildly optimistic, but I thought if I surrounded myself with like-minded souls, they'd be able to carry me along. Well, that was the plan, anyway. Finishing in one piece without soiling myself and before midnight was my more realistic ambition. We gathered round our man holding the 4:30 sign and I found myself next to a lovely girl from Ireland, Joanne. She was a rugby player and had entered on a whim — she'd only done a few months training, but she was thirty years old, naturally fit and wasn't carrying an ounce of fat with her. Another girl wanting to do 4:30 was a Kiwi running for the Asthma Society. Her mum had rung me on the radio to tell me all about it and of all the people in the marathon, I find myself standing next to her. It's that Kiwi connection thing.

We shuffled towards the start line, on the Verrazano-Narrows Bridge and then all of a sudden we were off, a band belting out the Frank Sinatra classic 'New York, New York' to get us under way. I always find the start slightly alarming. There are far too many people and it's very easy to trip over other people's feet or find that you can't get through a group because they're too slow and hogging the road.

However, it was a glorious day and a tug boat in the middle of the harbour was sending out a fountain of spray. I resolved that I'd started this bloody thing, now all I had to do was finish — come what may. I found the run over the bridge quite tiring. It's quite a steep incline to start with and the downhill run is always jarring on the legs. But a real treat lay in store. We came down off the bridge, round the corner and into Brooklyn — and there ahead of us, as far as the eye could see, were cheering Brooklynites lined three deep on the streets. The little ones were at the front, slapping the hands of runners as they passed by, while their parents held up banners for friends or general all-purpose signs for all the runners. Bands played, crowds cheered — it was exhilarating and inspiring and breathtaking (which is a bit of a bugger when you need every last breath you've got!) and I felt like laughing and crying all at the same time. This was what it was all about. This was the New York experience and it lived up to every single story I'd heard from old New York hands.

I high-fived the kids, smiled at those calling out my name, boogied to the bands and tried not to wince at the man who called me Cur. The weather was absolutely perfect, I was drinking Gatorade at every drink stop and I was feeling good. I'd lost my pace group — in the exhilaration of hitting Brooklyn, I'd either been left behind or I'd surged ahead. I'm thinking I was off the pace, as I never saw them again, although I did see Joanne from time to time throughout the race and it was great to see a friendly face — well, there were two million friendly faces. It was good to see a friendly face I kind of knew. The New York Marathon route famously takes in five bridges and five boroughs — Staten Island, Brooklyn, Queens, the Bronx and Manhattan. It's also known as a challenging run — you run uphill as you cross the five bridges and then it's downhill for at least a mile coming off each bridge and that's punishing on the legs. If you don't take the corners like a pro, you could easily end up running more than 42 km. And the last 7 km are also tough, as there are inclines for almost every centimetre of the route. They're only moderate, but for people whose legs are already turning to jelly after running for hours, it's a brutal way to finish.

However, the finish was far from my mind. I was taking this run step by step. We left Brooklyn and headed over the Queensboro Bridge. This one I found particularly tough, as the uphill incline seemed to go on forever. It's old and echoey and kind of surreal running across it, especially when you suddenly come to the end and there's a sharp dogleg taking you back onto the road, which is lined with cheering spectators. The spectators are something unique to New York. They are absolutely brilliant. It must be exhausting for them, standing in one place for hours on end to cheer on the runners, but they make the event. Throughout my run the 'Looking good, Kerre!'s and the 'What is today, Kerre? Today is your day!'s perked me up when my energy was flagging. The other runners were also inspirational. I passed a woman whose T-shirt proclaimed her to be a breast cancer survivor of twelve years; another young man had written on the back of his shirt: 'If you think this is painful, ask my mom about her chemo'.

And just as I saw my mate, Joanne, throughout the race, so too did I see a young blind Iraqi war veteran, who was being assisted in the race by two young women who were member of the Achilles Track Club. This is an incredible, non-profit organisation that was founded in New York in 1983 to encourage disabled runners to get out there and participate in long-distance running. There are chapters all over the world, including New Zealand, and they do an amazing job of ensuring that just about everybody who wants to run a marathon, gets the opportunity.

All of these incredibly inspiring people did a good job of keeping me on track. As the pain started to kick in with 10 km to go, I told myself sternly that I only had myself to blame. Any pain I was feeling was not as a result of injury or cancer, but because of overindulgence in food and drink and not enough training. A good telling off does wonders for getting you through the odd half hour or so. But by the time we reached Manhattan, I was feeling it. The Titirangi Tunnel Rats used to talk about having miles in your legs — that you had to have the miles in your legs if you wanted to run a marathon. And I knew I didn't have nearly enough miles in my legs. My butt hurt — that was a first — and my energy was gone, no matter how many power drinks I tipped down my throat. I was absolutely stuffed — and just before the 33 km mark, I began to walk. It was the first time ever I'd walked in a run — other than through the drink stops — and it felt like an admission of defeat. It also didn't feel any better and as I trudged along for ten minutes, I realised it was better to keep running and feel the pain for a shorter length of time than it was to prolong the agony by walking. So I cranked it up again and started shuffling towards the finish line.

Finally, we were into Central Park. The end must surely be in sight. But oh, no, my friends! Do not be fooled. You are still freaking miles away — 3.5 miles away to be exact. And miles suck. They don't click over with the same regularity as kilometres. The mile signs seem to take forever to turn up and you find yourself thinking that you'll never get there, which is most demoralising. I had a deep and irrational loathing of miles by the time I'd hit the gates of Central Park. However, despite the fact that you're in a whole other mind sphere when you're just minutes away from finishing a marathon, try, if you can, to enjoy the last long straight through Central Park — it's like running down a French avenue and it's lined with cheering spectators. And I did take a moment to enjoy this part of the run. And I enjoyed it all the more because as I was running along I saw a face in the crowd that I knew. There, standing against the fence, was Sean Fitzpatrick and his wife, Bronny. Out of two million spectators, I spot a couple of Kiwis. I ran up and they greeted me warmly and we exchanged hugs and Bronny said that they'd been wondering if they'd see me. And they did. It was most serendipitous and gave me a boost to get to the end.

As I jogged off, with their encouragement echoing in my ears, I knew my time left on this course could be measured in minutes, not hours. But there was more disappointment to come. As you head down towards 5th Avenue it seems logical the marathon should finish at the end of the straight. There's a monument to mark the end of the straight and if the organisers had any brains or sense that would be where the finish tape would be. But no. Round the corner, down another bloody hill, and then finally, there's sign saying we have just 300 yards to go, which cheers me up even though I have absolutely no idea what yards are, although I have a fair idea that they're less than miles. I see Gaz in the crowd taking photos and I cross over to give him a sweaty hug and then a few steps later I'm over. I've done it. The time on the clock shows just over five hours, but I know my time will be less than that as our blue group started so much later than the course clock. So I'm quietly pleased. Well, I would have been if I wasn't so stuffed. As it was, all I wanted to do was get the hell out of Central Park and get back to the hotel to get ready for our night out. I didn't want my photo taken, but I was very pleased to get my medal.

Volunteers handed me a heat sheet to wrap around myself and a bag of goodies, but I declined them. I was out of there and I had no intention of hanging around. Except that it seemed half the field was finishing at the same time as me. Although the marathon organisers had promised that a new and improved finishing area had been created to ease the congestion of past years, it was a nightmare. Literally thousands of us shuffled along on the narrow road, all being herded towards one tiny path that took you out of the Park. You couldn't cut across the Park and head out to the East Side, which was where I wanted to be. You couldn't bypass the baggage trucks even if you didn't have any baggage. It was a torturous shuffle to get out of the place. And as I was limping along, thinking how very foolish I'd been to discard my heat sheet and my goodie bag, like a ministering angel Joanne appeared by my side. She'd finished about five minutes before me, and someone had handed her two heat sheets. She passed one over and gave me a nut bar and then she vanished into the crowd again and that was the last I saw of her.

Eventually, after about an hour, I made my way out onto the West Side streets of New York, but I knew it was a long way back to the hotel. I fished my twenty bucks out of my pocket, which was now soggy with sweat, and stood on the side of the road, arm raised, to hail a yellow cab. I congratulated myself on my foresight, but as cab, after cab, after cab went past I realised that every other person in the marathon, along with their support crew, had had exactly the same idea. Fifteen minutes went by and I continued to stand there like a small round Statue of Liberty, my arm raised forlornly. It was getting really cold now and I was seriously hungry and fed up. Just as I was about to throw myself onto the bonnet of a taxi and demand that it take me back to the Bentley, I felt a tap on my shoulder. I looked around and a pleasant-looking man was standing next to me, shaking his head.

'You're never going to get a cab, sweetheart,' he said.

'But I just want to go home!' I wailed, feeling tears fill my eyes. I know I was being a wuss, but hey, I'd finished the freaking marathon an hour and a half hour ago. I just wanted a hot bath and a pizza. How hard could it be?

My new friend took me by the arm and led me into his shop, which was a running shoe shop. Hence his interest, I suppose. He gave me an energy drink from the fridge in the store, asked me where I was staying and told me the best way for me to get home was by bus. He consulted a bus timetable and then took some coins out of his till. He refused the $20 I offered him, and told the staff to mind the store while he walked me to the right bus stop. He waited with me till the bus came, which was only a matter of seconds, then explained to the bus driver where I needed to get off to catch the connecting bus. And with that, he waved me goodbye and disappeared back into his store. I was so dazed and confused I didn't get the name of the store, which is something I bitterly regret. I would have loved to have repaid his kindness by sending him a gift from New Zealand, but the next time I'm back in New York, I'll see if I can track him down.

My fellow passengers were chatty and friendly, and my bus driver went three blocks out of his way to deposit me on the right cross street so I didn't have to walk anywhere and run the risk of getting lost. I thanked him profusely but he shrugged and said there had been so many road closures all day, it didn't make a blind bit of difference. I

waved goodbye to my new bus friends and sat down at the
stop to wait for my next bus. I was so close to home now
I could almost taste the pizza. I was finally on the East
Side and it was just a simple matter of one last bus taking
me twenty-odd blocks and I'd be there. As I was waiting,
a very glamorous couple came out of their brownstone
building and sat down at the bus stop next to me. They
were heading my way, off to dinner at a friend's house.
The woman, immaculately made up and warm as toast in
a cashmere coat, had run a marathon back in the eighties,
so she was interested in my story and we chatted away for
a few minutes about our respective runs. Her husband was
getting impatient waiting for the bus, and as a cab went
past, he hailed it and decided we would all take the taxi
to where we needed to be. I remonstrated with him that
I was too smelly and sweaty, but they both insisted, so I
hopped into the front seat, they climbed into the back, and
seconds later I was back at the Bentley. They refused any
money, even though I tried to offload my sweaty twenty
to the cabbie and after much protestations of goodwill on
our respective parts, they went off into the night and I
staggered upstairs and ran myself a hot deep bath.

I lay there, thinking about my extraordinary day. I'd
done it. I always knew I'd finish it, even if I had to crawl, but
the time was fairly respectable, given my lack of training
and at least I hadn't embarrassed myself. The day had been
perfect, the experience something that would stay with me
for the rest of my life and then — the cherry on the icing
on the top of the cake — I had met some unbelievably
cool and kind New Yorkers who went way beyond the call
of duty to make sure I made it back to my hotel in one

piece. They were hospitable and generous and absolutely lovely. Meeting them was worth running the marathon. I wish now I'd kept the sweaty twenty as my lucky note, but again, I wasn't really thinking clearly.

I luxuriated a little longer and then I remembered my hair appointment. I rang the salon (from the bath) and they told me to come when I was ready, they'd be open for a few more hours and not to rush. So I wandered down to the salon, grabbed a pizza on the way, and let the girls untangle my sweaty matted curls and pamper me. By the time I got home to the hotel, it was nearly six and some of our team were just making their way home. Some had had to walk the whole way home, others had finished late. Blair collapsed into my arms as he walked through the hotel door. 'Even my hair hurts!' he groaned, before heading up to his room to put himself back together. We all resolved to meet in the rooftop bar of the hotel so we could toast one another and hear each other's stories before heading out to a flash restaurant, set up by New Zealand chef Peter Gordon, that was having a birthday party.

We were frocked up, absolutely delighted with ourselves and ready to take no prisoners in our assault on New York. Everyone made their way to the bar upstairs and Ange presented us all with a red rose each, part of the bouquet her partner Lachie had given her. Her run was particularly gutsy — a gnat's hair over four hours and she had been terribly ill in the days leading up to the race. She was on serious antibiotics, was throwing up for the first 10 km and had battled it out to finish, and finish in fine style. Everyone had war stories to share — Hils was bitterly disappointed because her aim was to finish in five hours and get her name in the *New York Times*. (All runners who make it in five hours or under get their name printed in the *Times*.) And although she was on track for three-quarters of the race, the last quarter damn near killed her. But as Gaz pointed out, given the operations she'd had on her legs when she was a child, she shouldn't even have been walking, far less running marathons. Finishing was a magnificent achievement in itself.

Kamilla said she'd burst into tears running down 5th Avenue and a number of spectators had asked her if she was OK. She called out that she was just so happy to be there, she couldn't quite believe it. Five hours 15 and she loved every minute of it. Nick couldn't be there. He'd had a terrible time — from the first drink station, he'd been unable to keep anything down. Wife Bindie had left him lying on the hotel bed in charge of the remote and had come upstairs to relate his story — and drink his share of the champagne. JM had probably the most dramatic run — scorching up the course, he was well on his way to doing a sub-three marathon, which is extraordinary given he'd only started running less than a year ago. He was sprinting through Central Park, with less than a mile to go, when he put his foot down and his whole leg collapsed under him. He had completely cramped up. The crowd gasped and a woman came forward and put a banana into his hand and told him to eat it. Another offered him an orange and a man started vigorously massaging his leg, trying to get some life back into it. He stood up and collapsed back down again, but with the help of his new friends he managed to get back up, and finish the marathon in just under 3:15. The last 2 km took him almost as long as his first five. It was great to share in everyone's triumph — Livvy and Geeling had had brilliant runs, Steven was a machine and Blair did exactly what he set out to achieve — and really we could well and truly say Mission: Accomplished. Especially in light of the fact that, because we'd all finished, we'd managed to raise more than $90,000 for the BCRT.

Those of us who were willing to kick on climbed into a couple of cabs and headed for Soho. You may have heard stories of Katie Holmes running the New York Marathon and heading out to her husband's film premiere afterwards in high heels. Oh, please! High heels? They were Kumf high heels, compared to what the girls from the Mission: Possible team were wearing. We couldn't believe all the fuss over Katie's run. You know how I said it's terribly poor form to mention how much pain you're in when you're running? It's also pretty poor form to disparage anyone else's marathon. There's an old adage that you can only be sure of two things when you set out to run a marathon: you won't be first and you won't be last. It's all about beating yourself, not beating other people. It's a personal journey, your challenges and triumphs are your own, not anybody else's — yadda, yadda, yadda. And I'm not disparaging Katie's effort, honestly . . . but really! Five and a half hours with all the help that she had? It was a good feeling to know that an old fat chick from the 'burbs like me had whipped her skinny rich butt. And now, having committed that to print, I'll await the Fates to dispense punishment for my hubris.

We walked into the restaurant wearing our medals and proceeded to sip champagne and mingle. It was a desperately cool restaurant. Fabulously specced out and a crowd of interesting and beautiful people who looked on in astonishment as we all worked the room. The first person I met was the son of an old restaurateur mate of mine in Wellington. There's that Kiwi connection thing again. The music got louder, as did the young Kiwis, and Gee and I decided that the two nanas would head off to a nice restaurant to have a meal before heading back to the hotel. And just as well we did really. The kids kicked on, slaying the crowd with their dance moves, and lurched in at about five. Two marathons in one day. And the press were impressed with Katie Holmes' stamina. Hah!

The next day was even better. The marathon was over and, although most of us had painfully stiff legs, we'd all come through OK. In fact, it appeared every marathoner — all forty thousand of us — had suffered in the quads. You could tell the runners from the regular tourists because we were the ones who winced every time we had to step off a curb and subway stairs brought groans of pain. We smiled at one another sympathetically and passing New Yorkers patted all of us who were limping on the back and called out congratulations. And as a real gesture of hospitality, all marathoners get to ride the bus and the subway for free in New York on the Monday. You're supposed to bring your medal with you to indicate you'd been a runner, but the stiff legs seemed to be just as much a certificate of authentication.

We wandered into Bloomingdales and a beautiful girl behind the counter asked us if we'd run the marathon. When we said we had, she cried 'Then I was cheering for y'all!' and threw her arms around us. She said she went out to cheer on the runners and didn't have anyone in particular to support so decided to cheer the overseas runners. And there were plenty of those. Her attitude was indicative of the whole city's. New Yorkers' participation in their city's marathon is phenomenal. It's extremely well organised (apart from the finish) and the goodwill of the people of the Big Apple makes it one of the most extraordinary experiences you will have in your life. Right up to the time we left New York, we were encouraged and supported in our achievement. As I was checking in my luggage (shockingly overweight thanks to Woodbury Common), the check-in clerk flicking through my passport said, 'You were only here for a short time, girl' and I said I'd just come to run the marathon. He looked up and said, 'Where's your medal then, girl?' I told him I'd packed it because I didn't want it setting off all the metal detectors and he held up his hand. 'Ah, ah. No way! You put that medal on girl, and you be proud. What you did was very special.' So he waited while I dug through my luggage and took out my medal and put it on. The security girl was much the same. She gave me a big hug and told me well done when she saw the medal and held it in her hand as I passed through the metal detector and showed it to her colleagues. This culture of celebration is a wonderful thing to be a part of. Can you imagine what would happen if you proudly wore your Auckland Marathon medal out as you pub-crawled up Ponsonby Road? If people didn't call you a wanker, they'd certainly be thinking it.

It had been a magical experience. The running of the marathon, the fun with our group, the kindness of strangers — it had been one of the best trips of my life.

GAZ

This is what it comes down to. Ten runners, five supporters and one coach in a very, very big city with a very, very long run! I admired those guys, they put their total trust in me through all those months of training. If you have never ran a marathon before, to choose New York is a pretty gutsy effort. With so many participants, you can't expect to run a very good time; runners are jammed shoulder to shoulder and nobody seems to want to be passed. Mind, that's not what you're there for. For most people, this is the only marathon they will ever run, so good on them. They should make the most of it and savour every moment!

I remember very clearly standing in one spot in the finishing chute for three hours because if I left it I wouldn't have a show of getting it back — someone would snap it up in an instant. I was taking photos of all the runners on struggle street; you could just see they wanted that 200 yards to go a hell of lot quicker. Next thing, who do I see jumping up and down, smiling, laughing and generally looking like a superstar? Our very own Kerre Woodham! It was the greatest sight and just goes to show what it's all about! That image will stay with me forever!

If you are ever going to run an overseas marathon, you must go with a group. The camaraderie in our group was just amazing. Everyone in the group got the support they needed from the others and there was a definite bond between everyone. This was the first time I had been involved in anything like this, but it will not be the last. I sometimes wonder if it was about the actual running or more about the journey to the race. I mean, the team could have been training for a bike race or the world Scrabble tournament with the same lead-up to the event: months of training in a team environment, fundraising for charity, having a farewell champagne breakfast and the host city embracing you with enthusiasm. What matters is what you learn along the way, whether it be that you never want to run again or that you discover strengths you never thought you had. You will take that memory with you for life. That's why I say that everyone has a marathon in them. The important thing is taking on something bigger than life and stepping out the other end. The marathon is just the tool.

chapter ten

Living, not just surviving

And now it's the start of another year. The New York Marathon is a distant memory and I've only just started running again. I went into a complete decline after I came home from New York. My enthusiasm for exercise, which was half-hearted at best leading up to the marathon, deserted me altogether. I was lethargic and lazy and apart from the dog walks, I did nothing. I've kept up the Pilates — I think I'll be doing that for life — but that doesn't get the heart rate up, unless Ree and I are rolling round the floor laughing. All the lovely dresses I bought for myself after the Auckland Marathon don't fit me any more — in fact, that's what got me going again. After the orgy of eating and drinking that was Christmas, I was down to two dresses that I could get into — love that Lycra! — and my seventy-year-old mother went home with two pairs of my dress shorts that I don't think I will ever fit again. She tried but couldn't quite hide the smug smile as she roared back to Hamilton in better nick than her daughter. I'm fatter now than when I first presented myself to Gaz a couple of years and two marathons ago and I can't quite believe I'm right back where I started.

Actually, I can. It's always been this way for me: blow out thanks to fabulous food and gorgeous wine; horrify myself with my excess and my inability to fit my clothes and get my act together all over again. I had fun blobbing out but now the party's over and it's back to pounding the streets again. Crikey, it's hard work too. It's hot and I'm heavy and there's pity in the eyes of passers-by again. The good thing is I know what I have to do to get myself decent again, and I know that I can and will do it all over again. But although my lack of wearable clothing has reached critical stage, for me it's not just about how I look. For me it's all about mental fitness. With the benefit of age comes the benefit of self-knowledge and I know that if I don't have a project or if I don't set myself goals, I start to pick at the fabric of my life and eventually it starts to unravel. I have the addictive gene running through my DNA and the Piss Fairy is always there, sitting on my shoulder, whispering evil temptation into my ear. You've probably met the Piss Fairy yourself on the odd occasion. There you are, planning a quiet Wednesday evening in with the kids while your husband is away on business and a friend drops round on the way home from work. A couple of hours later, you've got Bryan Adams on at full blast, you're dancing round the living room, you've sent the oldest child out for McDonald's and the two of you have even polished off the bottle of crème de menthe that's been sitting in the booze cupboard for the last ten years. A night like that is never planned, and is certainly not wanted, but when the Piss Fairy sprinkles his dust, you're goners. So I'm constantly battling the Piss

Fairy. He took the first decade of my adult years, I won back seven — and now we've reached an uneasy truce. But I know unless I get cracking and start on something that will consume my energy and require enormous amounts of self-discipline and mental toughness, the Piss Fairy will gain the ascendancy and I'll be history. That's why I decided to go to university to get a degree when I was 32. That's why I took up the liver cleansing diet and kickboxing and that's why I decided to run a marathon.

My Irishman often says to me, Can't you just be still? And no. I don't think I can. I have to be moving, I have to be juggling numerous different balls in the air, and if one or two crash to the ground, well, I'll just pick up another one. Although it's tough at the moment, I'm glad I'm back running. I'm going to try to drop some weight and run a decent half in the Auckland Marathon and Lavina, Lee and Mary are talking about doing the London Marathon in 2009. That's something to aim for.

The good thing about human beings is that we have free choice. If we want to sit at home and eat gorgeous food and balloon out to a super size, we can do that. Especially now there are fabulous clothes for the fuller figured woman. And if we want to be trim and lithe, we can be that person too. It just takes a bit more effort and discipline than it does to become a gourmand. Nobody can force you out the door to exercise. You have to decide you want to do it for yourself. Good luck if you decide to become a marathon runner. It will be one of the defining experiences of your life and mark you out as someone special. If marathon running proves not to be for you, do something else. You're healthy. There is no reason why you shouldn't undertake a magnificent accomplishment, especially when you consider all those women and men who would love the chance to achieve a goal but they can't because life has thrown them a curve ball. If you are fit and you are healthy, you have to suck the marrow out of life. At least once a year, you must disconcert your husband and alarm your children. That way you know you really are living and not just surviving. Once again, good luck and I look forward to reading about your adventures.

chapter eleven

Sharing the experience

I want to share with you the marathon stories of some of my friends and fellow runners. We all belong to that exclusive club of marathon runners, but our reasons for running are as varied and different as our physiques. When we were training, we all agreed that it was the personal stories we read of people just like us that helped keep us motivated and daring to believe we could achieve such a monumental physical challenge.

It's easy to make excuses when you're overweight, or you're a mum, or you have a demanding job — yeah, right. Read these amazing people's stories and then come back to me with your excuses.

Now — go write your own story. Good luck!

Craig's story

I like setting goals. In fact, I think the best way to get on in life is set a task, do it and don't look back. If you make a mistake, then learn from it and move on, but as they say, don't be scared to make mistakes. Hence, after running the Auckland Half-marathon in 2006 (and feeling like a sack of shit for three days afterwards), I decided, after far too many New Year's drinks, that I would run a marathon. As fate may have it, my wife's parents have some friends who live in New York and were visiting Auckland early in that year. Thus, a plan was hatched: I wasn't going to run any marathon; I was going to run the New York Marathon, the big kahuna burger of marathons!

I snuck into the field with a bit of luck and a friendly travel agent. I'd nominated a time that would give me a crack at being somewhere near the front group of the forty thousand participants. Then I started to feel sick. Was I serious? Could I actually do it?

I put my concerns aside and did a bit of training, but then I decided the best thing was to get some professional advice so in early June I went to Les Mills and enquired about top-notch running coach-type people. 'I need the *crème de la crème*,' I said. 'The best of the best.' Instead, they gave me Gaz.

My fears rose after our first session when Gaz said, 'There's a lot wrong with your running style.' 'You're joking,' I said, although I may not have been that polite. I've run for years and I've never had any trouble getting one foot in front of the other. I didn't know what he was on about. Sceptical as I was, I tried Gaz's approach — it's hard to explain on paper what the difference was, but it was more efficient and, hey presto, I was away. Perhaps, I thought, this guy does know what he's on about.

It was shortly after this that I got to meet the rest of the team raising money for the Breast Cancer Research Trust. They were a very friendly bunch, but also a very busy bunch. As a result, the whole group was rarely together on the designated Saturday morning running days — inevitably some people were away, hung-over or both. The team had a very relaxed approach to training, but I'm convinced this was the best approach and it is where young Gaz came into his own. He led by example on the drinking front and the team eagerly followed. He did, however, demand that people keep to their programme, but he did so without being officious. 'If you don't want to train, then don't,' said Gaz, 'you just won't get there.'

Quiet Fridays and early Saturdays became the norm and we ran round Ponsonby, Mission Bay and then headed out to the Waitakeres for some hard-core Arthur Lydiard-style mountain running. Gaz also decided to put the team through a beep test. I'd never done a beep test before, but once I finished it I realised that there were a number of other four-letter words that could describe the test better than 'beep'.

As the training regime kicked in I got fitter and fitter. Eight months before I started training, the thought of running a half-marathon was overwhelming; now I would casually run one before dinner.

Training basically grinds to a halt in the last week or two before the marathon, and it is recommended that you stay away from alcohol while you taper off. That might be OK for serious runners, but we just wanted to finish, not win the bloody thing! Still, I'd set myself a goal of beating 3:30, so I tried to stay relatively sober.

Before we knew it, my wife and I found ourselves in the Big Apple. This is a magical place and it was obvious that the marathon was a big event for the city. Everywhere you went there were posters and banners advertising the race.

As it turned out, running the marathon was probably the easiest part of race day. To say it's a mission getting there is a bit of an understatement. Due to the need to close off roads you have to be at the starting area by 7 a.m., some three hours before the gun goes off. I was up at 4 a.m., left the apartment at 5 a.m. and took a cab to the buses taking the runners across town. It's quite odd arriving in downtown New York at 5:15 a.m. and seeing thousands of people in shorts, T-shirts and running shoes, especially as there are also a lot of people spilling out of clubs and bars.

Once at the starting corral I ate and then went back to sleep. I was surprised to feel so calm, but I figured I'd done the miles so why worry; in fact, I was jumping out of my skin to run the bloody thing. After the inevitable queue for the toilet I was primed and ready to roll. I snuck a little further up to the front. You're not really supposed to do this, but it seemed to me everyone was and, hell, I'd travelled about as far as anyone to get there so I thought they could cut me some slack! While waiting in the throng of people I chatted away to all sorts of nationalities and took in the collective excited vibe. Everyone seemed to be thinking the same thing — we're here, this is our moment, let's do it!

The gun went off and three or four minutes later I was

over the line and on the Narrows Bridge amongst what seemed like millions of others. The running itself was reasonably flat, but it did take a while to clear the crowds and get a bit of space. Along the side of the road were two million people cheering your name (we had ours on the front of our shirts). This was cool to start, but towards the end I felt like killing the next person who yelled 'Looking good, Craig'. Bollocks — I looked like a bag of crap, but I appreciated the support. The race was actually quite a racket, with hundreds of bands and loads of other noise. The highlight for me had to be dropping down off the Queensboro Bridge back into Manhattan and hitting a wall of noise. At that stage I got a few tears in my eyes. It was truly something special; if you could bottle it, you could sell it for millions.

The only negative thing about so many people being involved in an event is that it's hard to spot, and be spotted by, your supporters. Although my location was being emailed via the transponder on my foot to my lovely wife, she had trouble tracking me down until the 23-mile (37 km) mark. It was fantastic to see her and she had tears in her eyes as we caught up. At that stage I felt very good. Unfortunately, less than a mile later I started getting cramp in my legs. I had wondered why people were offering runners potato chips along the way. I just figured it was fat Americans needing some quick snacks. As it turned out, I should have been eating those chips as the salt loss that caused me to cramp up would have been averted. The last few hundred metres were tough. I finally crossed the line in 3:26 and slowly walked amongst the crowd to get my gear and get out of there.

I don't think there are many times in your life you can say you're truly proud of yourself; for me, this was one of them. That night the crew got together in a bar proudly displaying their finishers' medals. I can't remember ever feeling so satisfied. Everyone in the team finished and we raised money for a very worthy cause. I really do think anyone can run a marathon, but there is no easy way to do it. You have to set a goal and do the miles, but the finish is certainly worth it.

Helen's story

What a year 2007 was! At the start of the year I was 23 kg heavier than I am now and had absolutely no desire whatsoever to run a marathon. As far as I was concerned, driving 42 km was challenging enough for me.

I had always played sport, but an overindulgence in food and wine ensured I was always well and truly nourished — a bit too nourished, it turns out. I saw a photo of myself and it looked like I had been pumped up. It was time to make some changes! I already knew what I should be eating, but actually putting it into practice was the tough part. With a little help from Weight Watchers and a lot of encouragement and support from my fiancé, I managed to drop around 20 kg by May of 2007. I felt so much better and exercise became a bit easier.

In May I changed jobs and starting working in the Auckland CBD. I went from being a secondary school teacher to a recruitment consultant at Select Education. With that came another change. I joined Les Mills gym and met Gaz. I thought maybe a couple of little exercises, nothing too strenuous to start with — how wrong could I be! Before I knew what I was saying, I had agreed to run the Auckland Marathon and join his running group on a Saturday morning. Me — in a running group — who would have thought? So, the journey began.

The first week we had to endure a beep test. It was like school PE all over again. Apart from the running attire they were all wearing, you would never have thought the people I was with formed a running group. I was expecting Lycra-clad gym junkies jogging around reception as a warm-up. What a relief, then, to find this encouraging, friendly and supportive group that were to become my friends.

We met every Saturday morning to go for a run, either in the city or in the Waitakeres. I actually started to enjoy it. We chatted about how our running was going, the successes of the week. We were running geeks! We laughed, we cried, we sweated (lots), we fell over. What a great feeling to be part of such a special group of people. The motivation, support and encouragement we got from being part of the team was priceless.

The day before the Auckland Marathon was a fundraiser for the New York team to raise money for breast cancer research. It was an awesome event for a great cause. We went for lunch afterwards and then the nerves started. Kerre decided pasta and a glass or two of rosé wine would be good carbo loading — not the most conventional method, but it worked (much to Gaz's disbelief!).

The day finally arrived. I was so excited. They say the hardest part of running a marathon is the training. It's so, so true! The run was a dream. I couldn't believe that I was actually running the Auckland Marathon. The running group was around the course cheering for me, running with me, cycling next to me. There are no words to describe the feeling of the run and crossing the finishing line. The only way to understand is to do it too!

We were all running the marathon for different reasons, but we all had one common goal . . . to cross the finish line with a huge smile on our faces. With the never-ending support of my fiancé, friends, running buddies and Gaz, I managed to cross the finish line with the biggest smile on my face in 4 hours 5 minutes. I loved it . . . I am now addicted!

The next plan is to do some duathlons, another marathon in 2008 and a half-ironman in January 2009 . . . three weeks before our wedding.

If you have ever wondered if you could do a marathon — you can. You never regret the things you do, only the things you don't. Have a go!

Hilary's story

I'm forty-three years old, Deputy Chair of The Breast Cancer Research Trust and Ecommerce Director of House of Travel. Until March 2006, I had never run anywhere in my life. A special friend, Annie Wilks, was rediagnosed with breast cancer in February 2006 and feeling particularly helpless about how to 'fix the problem' I enrolled in the Run2Heal 5 km run, which benefited the Breast Cancer Foundation. Later that year I became Trustee for The Breast Cancer Research Trust, a not-for-profit organisation dedicated to urgently finding a cure for breast cancer through radical and breakthrough research. The sense of urgency in the organisation is high, as breast cancer is increasingly becoming an epidemic in New Zealand.

When Annie passed away on 13 December 2006, I vowed I would do whatever I could to solve this horrible disease that affects one in eight women in New Zealand.

The Breast Cancer Research Trust was approached in January 2007 to be the beneficiary of the fundraising activities of a group of ten runners aiming to run the New York Marathon as the Mission:Possible team. There was one space left on the team and I leapt at the unique opportunity to combine my passion for travel, a strong desire to find a cure for breast cancer in my lifetime and the need to set myself a hugely challenging goal.

I am not a natural runner, having been born with hip problems that were controlled through an operation when I was six, which left me with metal plates in both legs and needing to learn to walk again. The marathon distance seemed quite daunting; however, I was surrounded by incredible support from a great team, trainer, support crew, colleagues, friends and family, and the other Breast Cancer Research Trust trustees.

Committed to running the marathon to contribute to research to ensure there is a future where women in New Zealand don't suffer the way Annie did, I was motivated through a training programme that had me running kilometres totalling the length of New Zealand! A slow runner, I took longer to cover the necessary distances than anyone else.

My job has me travelling regularly and fitting in five training days a week, full working days and travel proved a huge coordination exercise. Rest days were often filled with day trips to Christchurch and Sydney, which didn't always feel like rest. Over the ten months I ran in Auckland, Wellington, Christchurch, Sydney, Las Vegas, Berlin, St Petersburg, Moscow, London and Nice, with temperatures ranging from just above freezing to nearly 40 degrees. It's exhilarating pulling on your running shoes and jogging past the sights of these historic cities.

New York was everything I imagined when I took on the marathon. The city was alive with marathon fever and the team was buzzing. Registration at the Expo was our first formal step. We got our numbers, transponder chip and T-shirts, and wandered through all the stands, soaking up the atmosphere. Being part of a team all wearing matching jackets felt special. New Yorkers were keen to know who we were, what we were doing the marathon for, where we were from, and everyone seemed keen to talk to us.

When the day finally came, it was so exciting. My gear and power breakfast all carefully lined up, I was out of bed and ready within minutes of waking. On the bus to the start the team members were like school kids on an annual outing, laughing, joking, excited and playful. The only sober moment was when we crossed the bridge to Staten Island and looked back at the Manhattan skyline in the distance and realised just how far we had to run.

The start was incredibly organised, with runners divided into orange, blue and green. Sponsors ensured we were fed and watered with bagels, coffee, power bars, Gatorade and water. At 9.15 a.m. we were corralled into starting groups and nerves started to kick in. Layers of old clothing were shed and were picked up by volunteers to be donated to needy causes. As we shuffled towards the start line, the starter cannon went — a band was playing 'New York, New York' as we started to run — it was really quite emotional. Everywhere you looked there were runners of every age, shape and form.

By the 5 km mark I was in my stride. Each mile there was a water/Gatorade stop and I took some on board each time, indulging in a little walk through the station. The sun was shining and it was really beautiful, yet only about 14°C, so ideal marathon conditions. Right from the first bridge there were supporters everywhere cheering us on. The Mission:Possible T-shirts had our names printed on, and so the cheers were really personal: 'Go, Hilary' and 'Looking good, Hilary'.

I'd set myself a five-hour target as if you met five hours your name would be printed in Monday's *New York Times* newspaper. At 10 km I was still on track. At 8 miles (just under 13 km), we joined the other colour starters and went through Brooklyn. It seemed like every half mile there was a band playing uplifting music: at one point in Brooklyn it was a gospel choir, at another the NYPD brass band. It seemed as if the whole of New York was there to cheer us on, and I found out later there were over two million spectators.

At the 13-mile (21 km) mark my legs started to hurt and the Queensboro Bridge still seemed a long way off. I was still on track for five hours at the 18-mile (29 km) mark and was setting a steady pace, and then I just started to struggle. The pain seemed to start in my lower back and finish in both big toes. I started doing a bit more walking but quickly realised that wasn't a good move as getting my legs running again was quite difficult.

At 20 miles (32 km), we headed into the Bronx — not a tourist destination, don't go here after dark! They had a video camera and big screen and you could see yourself running down the road. I can promise you that was *not* a good look. I'd thought that when we got to the top of the Bronx and turned down 5th Avenue towards the finish line and the last 5 miles, I'd feel relief, but by then I was seriously slowing. I knew the finish line was on 59th St — we hit 5th Ave at about 135th St and the mathematician in me worked out pretty quickly we still had a long way to go.

By this time the personalised cheering was getting to me; I thought if I heard one more person saying 'Looking good, Hilary' I'd probably leap over the fence and hit them. Probably luckily for them and me, I didn't have the energy to do more than think that thought. Five hours had been and gone and my only hope now was to finish. We entered Central Park with 3 miles (5 km) to go. While the cheering was getting louder, my ability to put one leg in front of the other was rapidly diminishing. That last 3 miles seemed longer than the whole run.

And then suddenly I had 200 metres to go, and Gaz was yelling my name to take a photo, and I was crying with exhaustion, the culmination of the eleven months of training and the thrill of crossing that finish line. Tears were pouring down my face as a man put the medal round my neck and congratulated me. This was followed by a survival blanket and a plastic bag with food and drink goodies was shoved into my hand. I had finished in 5 hours 40 minutes!

Back at the hotel, we regrouped and shared stories. It's such an individual sport and yet I'm so pleased I did it with a team. Everyone had a different perspective and all had finished, which was a fantastic achievement. The sight of all of us drinking champagne, hobbling, laughing and congratulating each other was so uplifting.

Kamilla's story

So why did I run a marathon?

The last two years of my life could have been the worst two years of my life. I could have had children who behave badly, or have been a mother who constantly shouted at and/or ignored her children, or I could have blotted out the world with happy pills or alcohol. After all, my marriage had ended and I faced the uncertain future that inevitably results from that event. By I decided that whatever was coming, it was not going to get the better of me.

My first marathon, which I ran in Auckland in 2006, was purely selfish. I would turn thirty-five within a week of the marathon, and in the previous year I hadn't spent a lot of time on myself, busy as I was learning how to be a single-income working mother with two children, one a pre-schooler and one only just having started school. Committing to that marathon was the best thing I could have done! Admittedly my family and friends were only too happy to be supportive, helping with care and even coming on training runs. The whole experience had a positive effect on me, to the extent that, after crossing the finish line in tears, I famously said, 'You know, that really wasn't that hard.'

New York, New York — well that was a different story. First off, I had to find someone to look after the children for two weeks. Fortunately, good old (at 72) mum stepped in. Then I had to get to grips with leaving my business for two weeks just as we approached our busiest time of the year. My staff survived, my business survived, and I realised that other people can be extremely capable, when they are given the chance — thanks, girls. I still had a lot of business detail to plan before I went on my trip, but, hey, I was going to be doing it anyway. I also had to get to grips with the cost of the trip and when you're a single mum, every penny is precious. I broke down the total figure into monthly amounts and then justified it as my entertainment and clothing allowance (all of which I would redeem in New York!). Well, when you're running as much as we were and you wear a uniform to work, there is little need for much else.

The fact that we were raising money for research into breast cancer really touched me. My dad died from colon cancer. He was only fifty-four. I was only thirteen. I was forging new ground too, as far as our family is concerned. My mum is not at all athletic — I have never seen her wear trousers, let alone a swimsuit. I decided that I would do the run for my children. I want to live a healthy, active life with them. I want them to see me physically put myself out there.

You may well be able to imagine what Saturday mornings were like while I was training. I'd wake the kids up, then bundle them into the car — still wearing their pyjamas — and drive them round to their nana's house, where they would be deposited, cuddlies in hand, by 7 a.m. All this so that I could get down to St Heliers for a run with the team.

At other times I would take the kids up to the school, where I would set them to playing while I ran laps around the school field. And sometimes we'd all get active together, as I ran along the waterfront with the kids accompanying me on their bikes. Of course, more often than not, I ended up hearing the dreaded words, 'Are we there yet?' or alternatively, 'Mummy, I'm tired. Can you carry me?'

It was all so worth it, though. When I came back from New York and walked into the arrivals hall at Auckland airport, all I could see was their happy, smiley faces. It was pure joy. My five-year-old daughter later wrote to Santa and told him all about her mum's run. My son wore my medal to school for three days and told everyone that I had won the race — if only! Later he drew me a card to say how cool I was — the picture showed a long-haired lady running and another wearing a medal.

The run itself was amazing. New York knows how to put it on. The support on the street was tireless. When we started and the cannon went off, and Frank Sinatra's 'New York, New York' started playing, everything was electrified. It was like being fifteen and at your first New Year's Eve party without any parents.

There were a lot of laughs along the way, and a lot of moments that can still bring tears to my eyes today. Well, I am a bit on the emotional side! When we were running over Queensboro Bridge all you could hear was this amazing pitter-patter of feet. Then when we emerged from the bridge, from dark came light, from mesmerising shuffling came a surging of noise and cheer and people and faces, and happiness and emotion, and me. I started hyperventilating, but I put my head down, my iPod on, breathed and focused. And it was OK.

And then there I was at about 30 km sitting in a Portaloo, down some side street in that great city, giving myself a talking to. I had wanted to finish the race in 4:30, and I had stuck with the pace team for most of the first 30 km, but then I discovered that my tummy had other plans for me.

Needless to say the next 5 km took about an hour, but I am still so proud of myself for getting off that toilet seat and cranking out another 7 km on pretty heavy, stiff, tired legs and being able to keep up the pace till the end.

As I turned into 5th Avenue there was a very cool song by Pink playing on my iPod, and that was it — I bawled my eyes out for the length of the street. All I could think was I was actually here, running down 5th Avenue. This was for me, for my hard year of life and training, and for my children! Boy, I wanted to cuddle them. I was really crying, so much so that people kept stopping me to ask if I was OK. I was — I was just so happy that I was there.

The whole experience from start to finish was an amazing journey. I found out a lot about myself and my inner strengths. I was a little underprepared (which was my fault), but my mental discipline got me through. I made some fantastic new friends and I love them all. Nothing will erase the memories of what we achieved together. I don't think anyone could do this alone, and I had some wonderful support. Mel, in particular, was a huge support to the whole team and, one day, I'm going to do the same for her.

Lavina's story

I was six months pregnant and heavily hormonal when I first agreed to run the New York Marathon.

My regular running partner, Lee Taylor, easily ate up half-marathons, but had vowed never to attempt the 42 km. My neighbour, Mary Lambie, the most determined woman I've ever come across, convinced us both it would be an experience of a lifetime, and she was right, but we had just twelve months to prepare and, for me, six of those months would be consumed by pregnancy, childbirth and breastfeeding.

This would be my first marathon. I'd been jogging for years, doing maybe a couple of 40-minute runs a week, but I'd never competed in a running event, and rarely did I ever clock further than 10 km.

In January I gave birth to my second child, a month later we moved from Auckland to the Bay of Plenty for business reasons, and I went on my first run at Easter. God, it nearly killed me. I ran about 300 metres and felt as if I was falling out of my body. I remember stopping on the side of the road and breaking down in tears because I'd agreed to run the marathon, had paid thousands of dollars for flights, and couldn't even trot a few hundred metres without collapsing.

It took a call from Lee to sort me out. She emailed me a training programme and, despite the fact we lived 300 km from each other, we were determined to train together.

Lee isn't the type of person who stands for excuses. I told her my husband was working seventy hours a week; she told me to get up earlier. I told her my legs were sore, my body tired; she said I'd get over it.

I'm a sports journalist and I was in Auckland for work every second weekend, so we'd run together then.

At home I would get up at 4.45 a.m. before my husband Brendon left for work, just so I could complete my five-day-a-week training programme. Despite his busy work schedule, Brendon was brilliant throughout my training. Some days I'd say, 'It's raining, I might run tomorrow.' Brendon would say, 'You'll feel better if you run today.' Or when he got home and our kids needed bathing, feeding, reading to . . . he'd say, 'Off you go.'

The training wasn't easy; some days were certainly tougher than others. One day I was working in Invercargill when I was due to run 16 km. Outside it was zero degrees and the wind was howling. I remember losing the feeling in my nose and fingers, but I knew if I didn't run that day I'd be behind the programme the next, and I knew Lee was running in the North Island and would check up on me at the end of the day.

A few weeks later Lee came to the Bay and we hooked up with Kerre Woodham, who was working in the area. The three of us ran around Mount Maunganui. This was one of the most enjoyable runs of my programme. We scooted around the Mount on a typically spectacular Bay of Plenty morning — all of us working mums catering for the needs of our family and still finding the time to train. It was fabulous. My father used to talk about running being addictive, and it was on this occasion that I understood what he meant. That night I went to bed feeling a million dollars.

Some weeks later I ran 35 km, my last big training run before the marathon. Even though I finished it, the run took forever. That night I was covering a netball test between Australia and New Zealand, and my director called me to quickly get from one end of the court to the other to interview a captain. I just couldn't move. My legs locked up on me.

With the training complete the three of us arrived in New York. I fell in love with that city. It's so alive and active you can't help but be taken along for the ride.

The day of the marathon crept up on us. For me, the best part of the race was the start. Around 39,000 people all singing out 'start spreading the news' — finally, my dream of running a marathon was becoming a reality.

The race was tough, bloody tough. I felt fantastic at the halfway mark, but at 27 km I was struggling, wishing it was nearly over. My room-mate, Mary Lambie, had painted my name on my shirt so that the two million people watching from the course could yell out my name in encouragement. Sadly, it's not an easy name, but among the thousands of 'Go, Laverne's or 'You can do it, Lorna's the odd person got Lavina right and it certainly helped my cause.

I lost both my running partners along the way, which saddened me, because I was hoping to finish it with a friend, but everyone on the course is a friend.

I trained for a 4 hour 30 minute time and crossed in 4:08. I remember breaking down and crying, uncontrollable tears falling down my face. I did it. I said I would and I did it. I trained hard, despite the fact I worked, my husband was hardly home, and my kids demanded of me every day. I was so proud of myself. I don't think women are that proud of themselves these days. The feeling reminded me of both times I'd given birth and gone to bed thinking I'd done a good job — running the marathon is one of the few times I've actually patted myself on the back.

My biggest regret was that my husband and kids weren't at the finish line to celebrate with me — I craved for them, and next time I hope they'll be there.

Yes, there will be a next time. I need running in my life. It keeps me sane, makes me a better mum and gives me balance. Without it I get consumed by the petty things. When I'm running, I don't have to work hard at being happier or healthier; running takes care of that for me. It's also a facet of my life where I am my own boss. I have to get out of bed in the morning; I decide how fast I go, where I run, what distance.

Lee and I have both had babies since the marathon; in fact, we both got pregnant within a week of returning from New York.

A short while ago we both ran together . . . it was a year to the day after completing the New York Marathon. I know it won't be our last run together. In fact, Mary is already thinking London, and she's a very persuasive woman.

Lee's story

The rumbling was getting louder. I couldn't work out what it was. It was cold and gloomy running through the Queensboro Bridge. My knees were hurting, and I needed a distraction. I concentrated on the growing rumbling noise. And then as I rounded the corner in to Manhattan I realised it was the sound of hundreds of thousands of cheering spectators. Lee Taylor — this is your Olympics.

About a year earlier my husband suggested I run the New York Marathon. 'Why?' I asked. 'Why would I want to put myself through that sort of pain?' Each time I finished a half-marathon, I'd think, 'You'd have to be mad to do a full one.'

'I'll pay,' he said. 'Think of the shopping, the bars, the restaurants.' He'd had me by the time he'd mentioned the shopping. Okay, 42 km was looking a little less painful.

In another life I would have loved to have been an élite athlete. In this life I am too lazy. And I lack the talent (a minor detail). But I do have determination when I really set my mind to something. And I was looking for a new focus. At forty-one, I was still overwhelmingly sad that I'd never have another child. We'd had years of fertility treatment, and had been blessed with a daughter, Scarlett. She was desperate for a brother or sister, and Alan and I really wanted another child. But after three miscarriages and endless treatments, the specialist had said it was time to get on with the rest of our lives, and accept there wouldn't be another baby.

Running was something I was reasonably good at. I'm not fast, but I have endurance. I'd given it away for the years I was trying to get pregnant, and I was really enjoying getting back into it. But did I have the mental toughness to get myself through a marathon?

I decided to get myself a proper programme drawn up because I was having lots of problems with my knees. My friend Lavina and I shared the cost, and motivated each other when it came to sticking to the schedule. Lavina had moved to Tauranga earlier that year, but often came to Auckland for work so we were able to time many of our longer runs for when she was in town. Often I ran alone, but it was better when I had company. The companionship made all the difference when I was finding a hill too steep, the weather was too cold, or I just wasn't in the mood. Mary, who was also running New York, had an endless supply of witty stories to take my mind off the pain. I just had to grunt every now and then.

Kerre introduced us to the Titirangi Tunnel Rats, a group of seasoned runners who ran every Saturday morning in the Waitakeres. They were so generous with their knowledge, and it was great to hear all their stories and shared experiences. And it was also very refreshing to run a different route. If you always run the same track then your body gets used to it and you get bored.

The training was tough. Because I had a child and a full-time job, I'd have to get up at 5 a.m. to run during the week. It was winter. Some days there would be frost outside and I'd end up watching E! channel instead. By the time I'd caught up with Britney's latest drama it was too late to go for a run and I'd be grumpy for the rest of the day because I knew I should have hit the road. Or stayed in bed.

A friend gave me a book called *26.2: Marathon Stories*, which is a collection of individual running experiences.

On the days I really struggled to get out I'd read a couple of them, feel inspired and pull my shoes on.

I ran lots and lots of hills. It didn't matter how slowly I went. I'd go up one side of the road, down the other. Over and over. It made my legs really strong. Some days, to relieve the tedium, I'd pretend I was a famous athlete running a big event. Whatever got me through . . .

My knees were constantly sore. I had to ice them after every run, and had physio twice a week. Every now and then I'd get really disheartened because I could only manage the long runs if I took Voltaren first. Then I'd be limping round afterwards. I was seriously worried that I wouldn't even be able to line up for the marathon because they were so sore. After five months of carefully planned training I knew I'd put in the mileage. I knew my head was there, but I didn't know if my knees would hold out.

For race morning I had a carefully planned ritual. I got up around 4 a.m., had a shower, smeared myself in the gorgeous-smelling body lotion my workmates had given me as a good luck present and read the card they'd written (which meant I felt a bit of pressure). And lastly, but most importantly, I looked at the beautiful little book of photos my daughter Scarlett had made for me.

I hadn't had much sleep the night before — text messages kept coming through from New Zealand. But I'd read somewhere that it's the sleep you have two nights before the event that's the most important. Besides, the buzz in the city, even at 5 a.m. as we went to catch the bus, was so amazing it was impossible not to feel energised by it.

The marathon itself was fantastic. Over 38,000 people started in 2006 — only around 500 didn't finish. Around two million people gathered to cheer us on. There were bands playing. It was brilliant. To start with we were high-fiving spectators, waving, laughing, chatting. Then the reality of those long kilometres kicked in and we were a little more subdued. But as we came through the gloom of Queensboro Bridge it was truly amazing. Really uplifting. Strangers were shouting 'Go, NZ' (and some of them clearly had no idea what 'NZ' stood for).

I didn't feel any euphoria at the finish, just bloody relief. But the pride and excitement did come later. My husband and daughter shared it. Scarlett told everyone she knew that I'd 'won' a gold medal in the New York Marathon. One day I'll explain that everyone who finished 'won' gold.

Today, as I sit here writing this, my four-month-old baby is smiling and cooing in her bouncinette beside me. A few weeks after the marathon I discovered I was pregnant with Coco. There must have something in the gin — my running mate Lavina became pregnant at the same time.

Louise's story

I remember sitting at my computer late one night listening to the radio and hearing Kerre enthusing about the Auckland Marathon she had recently completed. I thought to myself, I'm going to be forty in 2007. I wonder if I could run my age in kilometres? On a whim I emailed Kerre to see how she had gone about working out a training programme, and to ask how much grit and grovelling would be needed to get my forty-year-old carcass around the course. Kerre replied: 'A group of us are going to do New York. Why don't you come along?'

The seeds of the idea had been planted, and as my husband will tell you, once I have a goal in mind, I'm a bit like a dog with a bone.

I've always been an active person. I live on a hill-country farm inland from Gisborne, and I love to get out there and climb the hills. I once was, in the days BC (before children), a keen mountain-biker and road cyclist.

Events conspired against my active lifestyle with the birth of my first child, Patrick. I had all the good intentions in the world, having jogged and walked during pregnancy. I figured I'd be back to all activity after the six-week check-up. But my baby didn't seem to be doing well. I couldn't feed him adequately, not even with a bottle. It turned out, after a lot of medical investigation, that something was wrong with this child's development. He was going to require my full attention and care, and numerous trips to Auckland for therapy, maybe for years.

My intended return to fitness was shelved, but with long hours of hard work, Patch improved. Eventually he could hold his head up, and then he could sit up, and by two and a half, although not yet talking, he could communicate by sign and was taking a few steps independently. By that stage I was pregnant with number two, delightful daughter Harriet, who did everything for herself with no help whatever: it was a revelation! Spurred on by little sister, our son began to speak clearly and to gain more independence. I bought a double buggy and started jogging. I progressed to quarter-marathons and even a half: it was great fun and I was hooked. I reconnected with girlfriends, also joggers, I had not seen for ages due to my tripping up and down to Auckland for three years.

But the week after our daughter's first birthday I took Patch to our GP. Patch was very pale, lethargic and, I suspected, anaemic. He had blood drawn, and I drove home to find the phone ringing. It was our doctor bearing the awful news that Patch had leukaemia. We were to pack up to leave for Starship Children's Hospital the next morning.

Family and friends swung into action: baby Harriet was collected by my mum and went to stay with her in Napier. Patch and I flew to Auckland, and husband Charlie had to remain at home to run the farm. I naively thought Patch would have treatment and be allowed home, but the treatment he required was very intensive, leaving him unable to make blood cells and very vulnerable to infection. The top floor of Starship became our home for seven months. Throughout that time I was totally focused on caring for Patch, but would frequently visualise myself running along the tops of green ridges on the farm. I was the most unfit I'd been in my life. I felt like a slug, but I was dreaming of running.

Our homecoming in September of 2004 was a great occasion. Mum had spoken to Harriet constantly about her family, and looked at photos of us every day. Harriet was very aware of who we were, and wouldn't let us out of her sight. She was walking and talking — milestones I had missed.

The slow road back to 'normal' life began. For many months after Patch's treatment we still had to be very careful about infection, and he was watched closely to ensure he remained in remission. We avoided contact with anyone other than friends who promised they were infection-free and would come to our near-sterilised home!

Gradually Patch got his strength back. He walked a bit further each day — to the mailbox, down to the horse paddock, down the road to see his cousins. Whenever Charlie could be at home I did the same — walking up hills, going a bit further each time. I was careful to walk for several months before attempting to jog, aware my bone density was probably not too crash-hot, since I'd been sitting on my butt for seven months.

Twelve months, almost to the day, after Patch was diagnosed with cancer, his appetite returned and the tube in his nose we had used to feed him was removed. His hair had grown back. He looked normal! School was looming in just a few weeks and, Patch having been socially isolated for such a big chunk of time, I was eager for him to start with his peer group.

It dawned on me that as Harriet was two, she could go to pre-school. I could get fit again!

What a change in circumstances! I could run. I could even go away for the odd weekend with mates and run in events. First I did the Tongariro Goat, which is a 21 km mountain run around a section of Mount Ruapehu. Then I decided to try to remember how to swim in order to do a small triathlon. Fabulous! Next, a friend and I took on a really big event, the Kaweka Challenge, and made it to the finish. What a sense of achievement that was.

As I jogged out the gate, the morning after my email exchange with Kerre, through the tranquil Gisborne countryside, an idea crystallised in my mind. Instead of poplar trees, I could imagine skyscrapers towering above me. In lieu of the babbling of the Waikohu Stream, I imagined cheering crowds. This would be a once-in-a-lifetime experience: the race of my dreams. I was going to enter the New York Marathon!

Once I had read every running book in the Gisborne library and had a plan worked out, it was a matter of following it. Not slavishly, but always with my goal in mind. The excitement of the destination was enough to keep me motivated throughout months of training completely alone on the farm and on country roads. After a nine-month build-up, a gestation of sorts, I felt incredibly fit and knew I would last the distance.

At the start of the race it occurred to me that each of those forty thousand runners gathered around me had been on their own individual journey to get there. During the weeks and months leading up to the race, we had been simultaneously running all over the face of the globe. Now here we all were, about to run in unison around the streets of New York.

Chatting to those around me I met a man from Arizona who was doing the marathon to mark his fortieth birthday, the same as I was. There was a woman with 'Running in memory of my sister Rose who died of breast cancer' in marker pen across her top. I saw blind runners, runners with all kinds of disabilities, each of us with a common goal in mind: to cross that finish line 42.2 km in front of us.

The most emotional moment for me was not the finish line, but after the first 2.5 km when we came off the stunning, mile-long Verrazano-Narrows Bridge into the screaming, hyped crowd in Brooklyn, who were reaching out just to touch the passing runners. That is, I imagine, the closest an ordinary person like me would get to the feeling of running in the Olympics. It was overwhelming, and the chap from Arizona burst into tears, as did I, and many others around us.

They say it takes a village to raise a child. It also takes a village to enable a part-time-working mother of two young children to run a marathon, and for that wonderful opportunity I'm indebted to my family and friends, in particular two very special friends, Lana and Neralie, without whom none of the adventures of the past few years would have happened.

I've been asked why I did the run. I guess the reason is that when I'm an old lady sitting in my rocking chair I don't want to look back and think 'I wish I'd run that marathon when I was young and had the chance to do it.'

I hope that everyone who reads Kerre's book will seek out and work towards their own New York Marathon, whatever it may be. The sense of achievement is amazing, and I have a big shiny medal to show my future grandchildren. I want them to think, 'Our granny was a go-getter'.

Martin's story

My name is Martin Tucker; I am a marathon runner.

Who would have thought a couple of words could change my life? Thinking back, I guess I should say thank you to the local social soccer group, who after one game told me I wasn't good enough to join their team. With encouragement (not nagging!) from my wife Kathy I got to talking to my good mate, Peter Fergusson. He suggested I come down to join him at the Takapuna Harriers Rat Race for a 5 km run and a beer, where the only competition is with yourself.

It changed my life. The runners at the Rat Race were so positive and supportive there was no way I wasn't going to improve, as my confidence grew and my title changed from disabled to runner.

The pavements of the North Shore have a fair amount of my skin on them by now. I was born with spina bifida, and with that comes a permanent challenge to my balance and coordination. Running really seemed to help both and the Rat Race women were always on hand with plasters. I reckon I should be entitled to a free coffee card at the local A&E, as I'm a frequent visitor, usually greeted with: 'Don't I know you?'

Reading the local rag one day I was interested to read about a group called the Achilles Track Club, which was helping a blind runner to compete in the New York Marathon.

Basically, the club encourages and supports people with disabilities to compete in mainstream events like marathon running. Since 1983 they have taken over 180 people with physical disabilities to run the New York Marathon. All of them completed the distance and received their medal.

Their motto is 'Failure is not an option'. I had completed a few marathons, but wow, New York, what an experience that would be.

Having been brought up mainstream, I don't consider myself disabled, so I had to ask Peter Loft from Achilles if I qualified. He took one look at me and said, 'Yes, Martin, you do.'

Jill Dickie from Pilates on the Move, my Pilates guru, started me off with strength training, the women from the Rat Race booked me in as training partners, and it was all on. I was so excited at the thought of running in the New York Marathon, and so humbled by the amount of support and generosity from everyone. Helen Bourne from Helen Bourne Office Services, Jill Dickie from Pilates on the Move and Martin Tregoning from Cue Sports Foundation provided the main funding for the Achilles group, enabling us to participate in this wonderful adventure. Their enthusiasm was inspirational, and I was just blown away.

When the day finally came, the training had been done, and there I was, just one among so many people — 39,000 of us — all with the same goal. My brother Andy and John, a volunteer from the Achilles Club New York, were by my side, and I can tell you now, the excitement and build-up is out of this world.

Suddenly there was a sea of people in front of me, it was cold, but there wasn't a doubt in my mind that I wouldn't complete. We'd had a pep-talk two days before the race, where we were told we would finish it. There are only two ways you won't get a medal, they said — if you're in an ambulance or in a body bag. I had no intention of being in either.

We ran through five boroughs, past two million people lining the streets, with a hundred bands playing. As I ran I heard encouraging words when . . . bugger! A groin strain started to form, and I couldn't run. A long time ago I had told myself it's 60 per cent fitness, 40 per cent head, so get your head into gear. Walking was my only option, so I started to walk. Seven hours and 21 minutes later, I finished the New York Marathon in darkness.

What a blast.

A piece of cake.

Thanks, guys!

Mary's story

Running the New York Marathon was a reward to myself. That may read strangely, the idea of a marathon being a reward; like treating yourself to some root canal work for a job well done. But a reward it was, and moreover a reward for running a previous marathon — the long and lonely slog of Rotorua, six months prior.

Rotorua was a miserable 4 hours 57 minutes, a wet nightmare, possibly the hardest mental and physical test of my life. But to complete it I had acquired 'fitness'. Since I had that fitness, I thought I may as well put it to a more glamorous and global use.

I ran the idea past my husband James. He readily agreed, which means that I must have promised to take the children off his hands for a morning when I asked him. Then I mentioned it to my friend and neighbour Lavina over a gin one evening, and we floated the idea of her doing it too. Imagine this scene — the two of us in a suburban kitchen, she pregnant and me with three kids under three, planning to run one of the great races of the world. But we are also Kiwi women. In no time we had flights sorted and a place secured in the biggest long-distance running race on the planet. Our dear friend Lee decided to come too, then we acquired a retinue of whanau, and soon we were a party of six.

New York was my third marathon. Ten years ago, single, childless and very much the career and party gal, exercise was my great love. That's when I first put the infamous Rotorua Marathon under my belt.

Fast forward a decade: I am housebound, busy but out-of-shape, with a pathological fear of becoming fat, slow and suburban, just a mother from the 'burbs in a domestic daze, wondering over the speed at which I had moved from a telly career to slopping around the house in my PJs, eating left-over roast dinners for breakfast and changing nappies with my eyes closed.

So I decided to re-run Rotorua, exactly ten years after I had first tackled it in my early thirties. Had my body declined post-babies? Could I get near my time of a decade ago? I had questions, but I also had answers — I needed a distraction outside of caring and fetching for the family. I'm a much better mother and partner if I have time away from the house, preferably doing something physical. I am a nicer person, fitter, too.

In retrospect, running Rotorua in 2006 was a truly barking endeavour. It put immense stress on the household. I wasn't single and fancy-free any more. I was already juggling dozens of balls in my life, and now I was adding a substantial training regime. But once my mind was made up, that was it. In April 2006 I was going to run Rotorua, come hell or high water. The way it rained that day, high water was the greater concern.

I employed the services of gun trainer Jon Akland, got myself a training timetable and began the ordeal of hauling myself out of bed on dank, dark mornings to pound the pavements.

My mate Lee lived around the corner. She is a far more natural runner than me, and set the pace in our joint training sessions. She had no plans to run a full marathon, however, and did not until we twisted her arm to come to New York.

The 42nd Rotorua race duly arrived. I was ready, more

or less. Irritatingly, but not surprisingly, I failed to better my time of a decade earlier. James and three small children had parked themselves along strategic parts of the course to cheer Mummy on, becoming as drenched as the runners in the process. I worry about what I am role-modelling to the children (let alone the extra parenting pressure I am putting on James) while I embark on these self-actualising endeavours — will it show them the value of giving life a go, or do I neglect them in mad pursuit of achievement? I suppose you are what you are.

So there we were booked for New York. I had no idea I was going to be asked to shoot an *Intrepid Journeys* episode in Iran for TVNZ just before the marathon. It meant being away from home for a month; in effect, arriving back in Auckland for only one night before jetting off again to New York. It also meant packing my running shoes and attempting to maintain my fitness in the middle of the Iranian desert, garbed in full Muslim regalia. It wasn't really the ideal build-up. I have seldom felt so guilty as when I hugged my children that one night back in Auckland, knowing that I would desert them again less than twenty-four hours later. But they smiled bravely at me, albeit a trifle wanly, as I fled . . .

What a great city the Big Apple is — all neon and noise — and we managed to take a few bites at it. Lavina and I shared a room; we shopped and drank and ate and shopped some more and then finally focused on the task at hand — running 42.2 km — or in American numbers, 26 miles, 385 yards — through five famous boroughs, in front of two million bystanders and a TV audience of more than a hundred million couch potatoes.

Logistically this race is astonishing. Think of the task for the organisers — you not only have to prepare one of the biggest cities on the planet for a foot race down thoroughfares normally teeming with traffic, but you must also wrangle the shunting of nearly 40,000 runners to the start line before the actual race even gets under way. We left our hotel at 4 a.m. and finally got to the start a couple of hours later. In zero degrees we waited for another couple of hours to set off, wrapping plastic rubbish bags around us to keep warm. But the combination of frosted breath and freezing limbs engendered a great spirit among the thousands of us waiting to get on the roads and test ourselves. Like cattle we were herded to the start, where Frank Sinatra was waiting to belt out his signature song; then we were off. The three of us ran together like a solid sisterhood for all of 10 metres before the race, the crowd, the confusion and the occasion engulfed us utterly and singly. The New York Marathon is an individual's race. You become part of a legendary occasion, and a player in a strange athletics dichotomy — there you are, struggling, jostling, fighting to survive and endure, with no-one to help you do that — but at the same time all manner of spectacle, including a hundred bands, is positioned en route to salute your lonely struggle, and to entertain the howling hordes of spectators who care not about you but about why you have come. They are there because they love the idea of this race; so did you, for the first few kilometres, before it got hard!

After a while, though, your thoughts transcend the fatigue and discomfort of a marathon. There is so much to look at, so many sights and smells, so much history and tradition that you are gliding past. You are running in the footsteps of others, and collectively they are giant footsteps. You become part of something that is infinitely bigger than yourself, but which needs you. You become magnificent.

Then, depending on how fit you are, that dreams ends with the infiltration of pain. It did get tough about 4 km from the finish. I spied Central Park, got my miles and kilometres muddled up, and thought I was a lot closer to the end than I was. And Central Park is hilly! It's up hill and down dale, a grim slog for a runner at the end of a race. With each corner I thought 'This is it; I'm there!' — but no, there was another corner ahead, and another and another.

Finally it was over. Who should be there, waiting patiently, but Lavina. She had come in a good half hour ahead of me, but waited, in the true spirit of mateship, to see me fall over the finish line. We clutched each other tight, and hobbled to collect our small bags of belongings and began the calls home. James had been following my progress thanks to the wonders of GPS technology, which informed him via e-mail, every 5 km, how I was doing. He knew my official time before I did. On the cellphone I heard Grace say, 'Mummy, did you win?'

'Yes, darling,' I said, through a vast, warm, weary fog, 'Yes. Mummy won. And now she's coming home.'

Tina's story

In 2007 I was lucky enough to meet Kerre Woodham, after my first marathon. As the conversation unfolded, she asked me if I would mind writing a piece on what inspired me to run a marathon.

It had always been a long and distant dream of mine to run a marathon, which seemed unreachable until I accidentally entered the Auckland Marathon. That's where it all started . . .

The one thing that truly inspired me was me. I suffer from depression and I need to find new ways to cope with the challenges life puts in front of me. Like many people, I have a big heart and a sensitive one at that, which would send my emotions into overdrive. What I needed was to find my confidence again and the opportunity came when I mistakenly filled out an entry form for the full Auckland Marathon, instead of the Half.

I decided to turn this into a positive, and found a personal trainer, Claire, who has since become a good friend. I was worried about my size-18 frame and big boobs, but with Claire's cool attitude and encouragement I embarked on a long, hard, four-month training programme. I ran every training run by myself and after my long runs I would text Claire with my progress. It was almost always *Shit that was goddam hard, mate.*

In the beginning, I would get embarrassed when a group of teenagers would drive by, toot and give me the fingers. But me being me, I'd give them the fingers back, followed by a few choice words and yes, it felt good. On the harder runs, I was lucky to have a friend I could call on for some words of encouragement and she would always come up trumps. Thanks heaps, Trace, you helped make it happen for me.

There were days when I really had to dig deep, and I started to realise I wouldn't be able to complete the whole distance without walking, so my focus and goal changed from running the whole way to running to the water stops, and then walking for five minutes after each stop. This was a much more realistic goal and became my focus.

With support and encouragement from my devoted husband and sweet, cool comments from my children — Mum, you've lost weight — I got there.

On 28 October 2007, I was on the start line of something I had always thought would be unreachable for me. Five hours and 36 minutes later I had finished, boobs over the pavement and all. I had achieved that long and distant goal.

The depression hasn't gone, but the *knowing I can do it* attitude has strengthened my belief in myself. I've set myself another goal, to compete in the Rotorua Marathon, and to enter a half-ironman event before I'm forty. Some people might laugh at me, toot, and show me two fingers, but I don't give a damn, because this is about me, and only me. Big girls *can* run marathons.

Appendix 1
A marathon training programme for beginners

The following is a general marathon training programme for beginners, developed by Gaz Brown. The numbers indicate the time (minutes) that should be walked (W) or run (R) on each day.

Anyone who is taking up exercise for the first time, or after a long gap, should consult their doctor first. Would-be marathon runners are strongly advised to get professional advice, especially if they start to have difficulties, such as knee, hip or foot problems.

Correct footwear is essential for anyone undertaking any distance running. Go to a sports shoe store that can analyse your running gait to help you choose the most appropriate shoes. If you have problems, then consider visiting a podiatrist, who will be able to give you a more detailed examination and, if needed, can supply you with corrective insoles for your shoes.

Phase 1
Phase 1 of the training programme is designed to slowly build up your base fitness. This is designed for people who have been doing very little aerobic exercise, which is why you do a lot of walking and only a small amount of running. The programme is designed to get you used to spending time on your feet. Although you may think you can go faster or further than listed, please do not attempt this, as you increase your risk of developing an injury — and then you will have to take time off and start all over again!

	Mon	Tues	Wed	Thurs	Fri	Sat	Sun
Week 1	—	W20	—	W20	—	W15, R5	—
Week 2	W20	W20, R5	—	W15, R5	—	W15, R5	—
Week 3	W5, R5	W15, R10	—	W15, R5	—	W15, R5	—
Week 4	W5, R5	W20, R5	—	W15, R5	—	W20, R5	—
Week 5	W5, R5	W20, R5	W10, R10	—	W10, R10	—	W15, R10
Week 6	R10	W20, R10	—	W20, R10	—	W20, R10	—
Week 7	W15, R5	W20, R10	—	W20, R10	—	W20, R10	—
Week 8	W10, R10	W15, R15	—	W20, R10	—	W15, R15	—
Week 9	W10, R10	W10, R20	—	W15, R15	—	W10, R20	—
Week 10	W10, R10	W10, R20	—	W10, R20	W10, R10	W10, R20	—
Week 11	W5, R15	W5, R25	—	W10, R20	W5, R15	—	W10, R10
Week 12	W5, R25	—	R30	W5, R15	R30	—	W5, R15
Week 13	R30	—	R30	R20	R30	—	R20
Week 14	R30	—	R30	R20	—	R30	R20
Week 15	R30	—	R30	R30	—	R20	R20
Week 16	—	R30	R20	—	R30	R30	R15

Phase 2

Phase 2 of the marathon programme is where you start to build up your mileage and get time on your legs. This time it's all about running — there is no walking involved. Again, don't go for longer than listed in the chart, and make sure you use the rest days. If you like, go for a bike ride or a swim on the rest days — just don't go for a run; your body needs the time to recover.

	Mon	Tues	Wed	Thurs	Fri	Sat	Sun
Week 1	30	—	30	—	35	25	40
Week 2	—	25	40	—	30	25	30
Week 3	—	35	30	—	30	25	50
Week 4	—	20	—	35	—	20	40
Week 5	—	40	20	—	45	20	60
Week 6	—	40	20	—	50	20	50
Week 7	—	30	50	—	50	20	70
Week 8	—	40	50	—	50	20	30
Week 9	—	50	40	—	60	20	80
Week 10	—	30	55	30	55	—	70
Week 11	—	60	35	60	40	—	90
Week 12	—	65	40	30	40	—	80

	Mon	Tues	Wed	Thurs	Fri	Sat	Sun
Week 13	—	60	30	50	35	—	100
Week 14	—	70	40	60	40	—	90
Week 15	—	70	30	60	35	—	110
Week 16	—	70	40	70	30	—	100
Week 17	—	70	35	70	35	—	120
Week 18	—	85	40	75	40	—	110
Week 19	—	80	45	70	40	—	130
Week 20	—	80	40	75	25	20	120
Week 21	—	85	35	75	20	20	140
Week 22	40	80	40	40	35	—	130
Week 23	40	90	40	90	40	—	150
Week 24	—	90	40	90	40	—	60
Week 25	40	—	40	30	—	60	20
Week 26	40	20	10	—	—	—	Race Day

Appendix 2

Kerre's marathon training programme

Kerre Woodham's training schedule as developed by Gaz Brown. Kerre had some base fitness, as she walked her dog every day. That, and her determination and willingness to consult specialists when she struck a problem, meant she was able to tackle this condensed marathon training programme.

MON	TUES	WED	THURS	FRI	SAT	SUN
			MAY 2006			
					27 run 15 min	28
29 run 10 min	30 run 10 min	31 —				

MON	TUES	WED	THURS	FRI	SAT	SUN
			JUNE 2006			
			1 run 15 min	2 —	3 run 30 min	4 —
5 run 30 min	6 —	7 run 30 min	8 run 20 min	9 —	10 run 30 min	11 run 20 min
12 —	13 —	14 run 30 min	15 run 25 min	16 run 50 min	17 —	18 run 40 min
19 run 20 min	20 —	21 run 45 min	22 run 20 min	23 run 60 min	24 —	25 run 20 min
26 —	27 run 35 min	28 —	29 run 20 min	30 run 40 min		

JULY 2006

MON	TUES	WED	THURS	FRI	SAT	SUN
					1 —	2 run 30 min
3 run 50 min	4 —	5 run 50 min	6 run 20 min	7 run 70 min	8 —	9 run 40 min
10 run 50 min	11 —	12 run 50 min	13 run 20 min	14 run 30 min	15 —	16 run 50 min
17 run 40 min	18 —	19 run 60 min	20 run 20 min	21 run 80 min	22 —	23 run 30 min
24 run 55 min	25 —	26 run 30 min	27 run 55 min	28 run 70 min	29 —	30 run 60 min
31 run 35 min						

AUGUST 2006

MON	TUES	WED	THURS	FRI	SAT	SUN
	1 —	2 run 60 min	3 run 40 min	4 run 90 min	5 —	6 run 65 min
7 run 40 min	8 —	9 run 30 min	10 run 40 min	11 run 40 min	12 —	13 run 60 min
14 run 30 min	15 —	16 run 50 min	17 run 35 min	18 rest; walk dog	19 fly to Blenheim, approximately 4 p.m.	20 Woodbourne Half-marathon; start 10 a.m.
21 arrive home; rest	22 rest; walk dog	23 rest; walk dog	24 rest; walk dog	25 run 30 min	26 —	27 run 70 min
28 run 40 min	29 —	30 run 60 min	31 run 40 min			

SEPTEMBER 2006

MON	TUES	WED	THURS	FRI	SAT	SUN
				1 run 90 min	2 —	3 —
4 run 80 min	5 run 45 min	6 run 70 min	7 run 40 min	8 —	9 run 130 min	10 —
11 run 80 min	12 run 40 min	13 run 75 min	14 run 25 min	15 —	16 run 120 min	17 —
18 run 85 min	19 run 35 min	20 run 75 min	21 run 20 min	22 run 20 min	23 run 140 min	24 run 40 min
25 run 80 min	26 run 40 min	27 run 40 min	28 run 35 min	29 —	30 run 130 min	

OCTOBER 2006

MON	TUES	WED	THURS	FRI	SAT	SUN
						1 run 40 min
2 run 90 min	3 run 40 min	4 run 90 min	5 run 40 min	6 —	7 run 150 min	8 —
9 run 90 min	10 run 40 min	11 run 90 min	12 run 40 min	13 —	14 run 60 min	15 run 40 min
16 —	17 run 40 min	18 run 30 min	19 —	20 run 60 min	21 run 20 min	22 —
23 run 40 min	24 run 20 min	25 run 20 min	26 —	27 —	28 —	29 The Big Race

Appendix 3

Well-known marathoners

Running a marathon is not just for athletes. Here is a list of some of the better known people who have run marathons.

Name	Event	Time
Lance Armstrong*	New York City Marathon	2:59:36
George W. Bush	Houston Marathon	3:44:52
P. Diddy (Sean Combs)	New York City Marathon	4:14:54
Al Gore	Marine Corps Marathon	4:58:25
Katie Holmes	New York City Marathon	5:29:58
David Lee Roth (from Van Halen)	New York City Marathon	6:04:43
Bjorn Ulvaeus (from ABBA)	Stockholm Marathon	3:23:54
Oprah Winfrey	Marine Corps Marathon	4:29:20

*Lance said that running the marathon was tougher than riding the Tour de France!

Appendix 4

Resources

The Internet is a great place for information about running in general and marathons in particular. Here is a list of websites that I found useful:

www.archillestrackclubnz.org.nz

www.aucklandmarathon.co.nz

www.bodyneed.co.nz

www.coolrunning.com

www.getrunning.co.nz

www.mapmyrun.com

www.physiopilates.co.nz

www.taupohalfmarathon.org.nz

www.ymcamarathon.org.nz

Books:

26.2: Marathon Stories, Kathrine Switzer and Roger Robinson, Madison Press Books, Toronto, 2006.

Going the Distance, Tracey Richardson, Random House, Auckland, 2005.

Lore of Running, 4th edition, Tim Noakes, Oxford University Press, Southern Africa, 2003.

Ultra Marathon Man, Dean Karnazes, Penguin, New York, 2005.